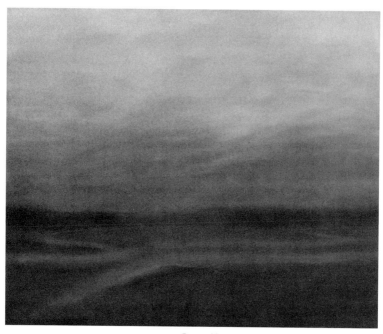

Cover Artwork: "Convergence"
Original: oil on canvas, 30" x 36"
© Sande Waters, www.sandewaters.com

The FAST Way to Heal for Life

The Healing Power is Within

"Our natures are the physicians of our diseases."
~ Hippocrates (460 B.C.)

Halanna Matthew, Ph.D.

Robert D. Reed Publishers   •   Bandon, OR

Robert D. Reed Publishers
P.O. Box 1992
Bandon, OR 97411
Phone: 541-347-9882; Fax: -9883
E-mail: 4bobreed@msn.com
Website: www.rdrpublishers.com

Cover Designer: Cleone L. Reed
Cover Artist: Sande Waters
Photographers: Aeron Matthew, Melissa Matthew, Cleone Reed, and some from www.morguefile.com: Earl53, Matthew Hull, Gracey, Jusben, and Zandert
Illustration: "How Disease Is Created Tree" original artist unknown, recreated by Cleone Reed
Book Designer: Corryn Hurst

ISBN 13: 978-1-934759-16-5
ISBN 10: 1-934759-16-3

Library of Congress Number: 2009923644
Manufactured, Typeset, and Printed in the United States of America

NOTE TO THE READER

It is the author's intention to provide true knowledge about healing through optimum nutrition, fasting and purification, exercise, sleep, rest, sunlight, pure water, etc.

However, if you have any health issues, obesity, or on medication, it is advisable to seek individualized care by a doctor or health institution mentioned in this book, or one that understands nutrition and fasting of your choice.

Symbols give meaning to our lives and those used in this book are forms of artistic expressions of healing.

THE FAST WAY TO HEAL FOR LIFE

"To die young as late as possible."
– Ashley Montague

DEDICATION

I dedicate this book to my son Jarome and his wife Felisha, my daughter Melissa and grandson Aeron, for their loving support and encouragement in believing in me as parent and friend and persevering with their health despite years of opposition. Without their help this book would not have been possible.

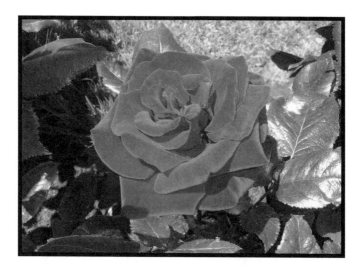

ACKNOWLEDGMENTS

I am most grateful to Dr. Herbert Shelton, who was my first teacher. In 1969 when I first wrote to him about my sick child he replied immediately with great concern, and with his suggestions the child was well in a short time.

My gratitude also goes out to my friends and mentors, the late Drs. Gerald Benesh and William Esser, who were so patient while I was raising a family and combating world opposition, who replied to all my queries with deep concern, and who encouraged me to continue my studies and to write books.

In recent times I am most grateful to Dr. David J. Scott for his timeless wisdom, and for replying to my telephone calls and answering all my questions with compassion. His kindness will be always remembered.

TABLE OF CONTENTS

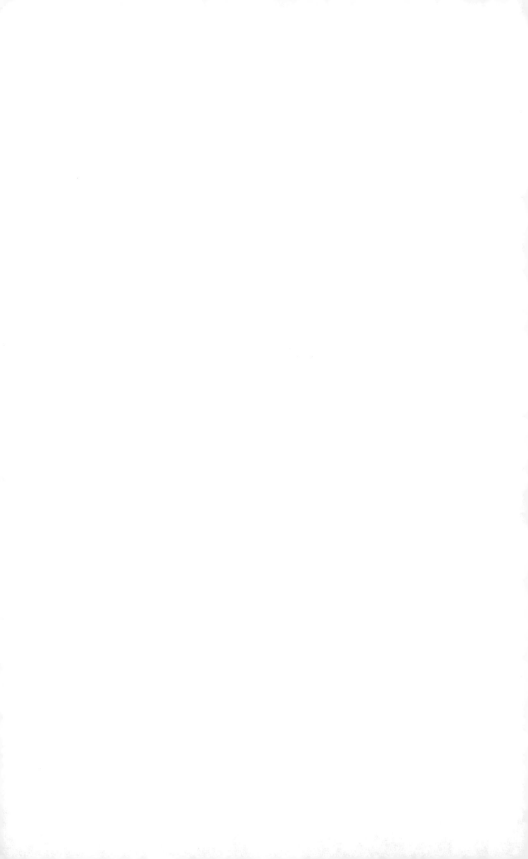

FOREWORD

The profound wisdom designed into the fabric of life is unfathomable except to the wisdom of understanding that life is self-healing, self-repairing and self-perpetuating. To my mind this can only be assigned to the wisdom of design. Such a magnificent design demands a designer of infinite wisdom that can only be explained by a God of infinite wisdom.

All the egocentric understanding of science which is frequently tremendous in scope but never represents anything but discovery of the designs in nature and that only, which is allowed to be discovered one tiny fragment at a time.

Design genetics has made it possible to perpetuate life in its infinite form through thousands of years in exact replications until modern man has discovered how to totally derange this profound genetic system by his warped genius for greed by treating symptoms, foods, water, air, etc. with toxic agents called medicine, preservatives, chemical fertilizers, purifiers, etc. As a result of the total toxic infusion of every part of our environment disease causes pervade our universe. Diseases practically unknown one hundred (100) years or more ago are now pandemic. Major diseases in the past were mostly traceable to hygiene sources. Now, however, diseases such as cancer and degenerations in general are tremendously accelerated to epidemic proportions by environmental chemistry, mal-metabolism of food, plus remedies such as toxic drugs.

Reversal of disease on the other hand is mostly possible and is allowed by natural law. But once advanced, broken-down health has developed, one's personal health must now be constantly maintained by continued obedience to one's personal mortal limitations and tolerances also under natural law.

Every single function of life comes built into every single living cell of life.

Magnify that by trillions of cells in every human body and then organize these cells into specialized tissues and organs; now you have one completely profound human organism perfectly regulated from inside. That total organism through its brain is in constant communication and control of every one of those trillions of cells. This whole automated system never for one moment sleeps or rests. All this control is carried on under such a complex computerized communication system called the brain which then in turn will assign priorities of importance, intended by design to carry to completion, every regulatory control for every single need for preserving, repairing, protecting, healing and regenerating the organism. Of course our personal and individual responsibilities necessitate that we act with intervention in life threatening emergencies. In most cases health problems can be resolved to recovery within the natural laws of our design nature.

I believe Halanna Matthew has brought together from the best resources in the world inspirational teaching, which can guide you with confidence and trust, to the care for life's needs by healing through fasting and natural garden nutrition with the opportunity to direct and guide your body back to health by healthful means. These means are consistent with the principles built into life. Of course there is one major proviso meaning if you are not widely experienced and trained you must choose to follow the guidance of one who is. This person should be qualified by training and experience, to understand evolution of pathology, and then additionally qualified by modern science to confirm the progress one is making.

Doctor Halanna Matthew has done an excellent work in this writing to accomplish this goal and destination. Certainly, she has earned and needs to be given deserved acclaim.

Dr. D.J. Scott, D.M., D.C., LL.C.
17023 Lorain Avenue
Cleveland, Ohio 44111

Rainbow

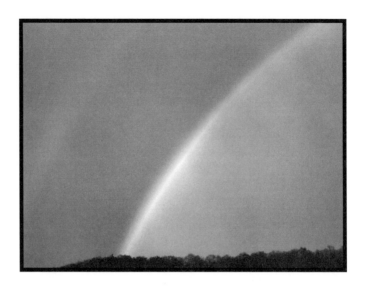

Hope - Promise

INTRODUCTION

It is as natural to be well as it is to be born.

OLD AGE IS INEVITABLE; DISEASE IS NOT

This book is about fasting and rejuvenation: the ultimate healing experience.

This ancient healing practice provides powerful transformation for healing physically, emotionally, mentally and spiritually. Cleansing the mind, body and spirit has been neglected for decades.

The practice of fasting to release toxins, to rest and to heal is powerful.

As one reads in this book the testimonies of those who have experienced the rewards of fasting, one will become convinced that:

- There is no other method of healing that compares to the outstanding results visible in a very short period of time through fasting.

- The miracles that occur through fasting, as well as the discovery of the primary prerequisites and truths to achieving and maintaining perfect health for the rest of life, are found in this book of wisdom.

- With our polluted environment, processed foods, stress, harmful addictions, wars, unrest and crime, it is almost necessary for the world to consider fasting as the most efficient solution, resulting in purification, healing and peace.

- This is prevention at its highest level.

- This is healing the entire human organism and the environment.

- True Health Care is each person caring for his body, mind and spirit.

By living according to the laws of nature, individuals can become productive and attain longevity as well as a quality of life without deterioration. By removing the cause of disease, usually the result of unhealthy living, the body heals itself. Proper health care does not require the ingestion of poisonous substances. Whereas allopathic medicine treats the symptoms of disease, the natural doctor focuses on allowing the body's innate wisdom and healing powers to work dynamically on behalf of the organism. To "leave it alone" means to not interfere with the body's own innate intent. With this approach, the organism has a chance to restore balance and eliminate toxins and conditions that may have caused sickness.

The best approach to health is to educate more and medicate less, so that individuals understand the nature of disease and learn how to remove the cause naturally. In doing this, the organism has a chance to remove the immediate cause of disease and to terminate the abnormal processes properly. To maintain and restore health and to prevent disease means to supply the organs with the essentials of health and to eliminate all harmful influences.

Fasting, also known as a physiological rest, is a time of change. There is no therapeutic method of healing that brings more transformation to the body, mind and spirit than taking a break away from food, thus allowing the body to rest.   In a state of rest the body is able to expel long-retained waste and to heal itself. During a fast the body may experience momentary weakness and tiredness. However, upon completion of the fast, the body is strong and vitally alive, and will remain so provided constructive habits are maintained and a healthy mode of living practiced.

The Sun

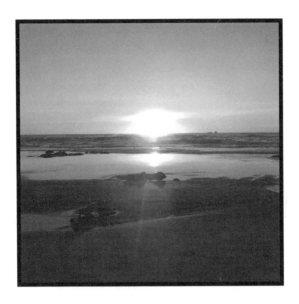

Warmth - Nourishment

THE FAST WAY TO HEAL FOR LIFE

...and you will be like a watered garden,
like a flowing spring whose waters never run dry
– Isaiah 58:12

When you stop eating you become strong and health returns.

Chapter I

THE PHYSIOLOGICAL REST

To fast on water only is remedial practice. This means that the disease that needs to be cured is the remedial action that restores health. The voluntary abstinence from food, while resting and drinking pure water as a method for eliminating disease, is as old as life itself. During the fast the innate power of healing within each organism repairs and remedies the sickness. Dr. Albert Schweitzer called this defense mechanism "your doctor within.

> "To fast when ill is the manna of health as it purifies the body, mind and spirit. Fasting restores homeostasis." The fast is the key to eternal youth, the secret of perfect and permanent health … It is nature's safety-valve, an automatic protection against disease." (Sinclair, p.25)

> "For ten or fifteen years…she had been a bed-ridden invalid … suffered from sciatica, acute rheumatism …

chronic intestinal trouble … intense nervous weakness, melancholy and chronic catarrh, causing deafness: she had abstained from food for eight days; she had cured herself by a fast." (Sinclair, p. 19)

WHAT IS HEALTH

We must eat to live, drink to live, breathe to live, exercise to live, and sleep to live.

The word health is derived from the Anglo-Saxon word meaning "whole" or "wholeness." There can be a contradiction with this meaning because some individuals will say they are healthy except for their arthritis, or others will say they are well except for their pain, or others will have been born with defects, or missing parts. Health is more than the absence of the symptoms of disease. Health is a state of positive well-being that is noticed by a constant state of euphoria and aliveness. People enjoying this high level of health are few in today's world.

Health is a state of soundness and integrity of the organism, vigor and efficiency of function in the entire body, including excellent mental faculties. Much of this is inherited and also created by how one lives.

"Health manifests itself by such a feeling of tone in the entire being that the body glows with it and bespeaks it at every turn. There is clearness and sparkle to the eyes, clearness and fine color to the skin, vigor of activity and bounce to the step, and an evident feeling of joy of living that is infectious." (Dr. Herbert Shelton, *Health Review*, 1979, p. 1)

Sometimes this pristine vigor and wellness is visible in young children. It is also noticed in young animals as they play and frolic. This vitality and zest for life is possible to human beings throughout most of their lives when living according to the laws of nature.

"When we see children who are clear of the eye, with fair radiant skin, who are full of life, are active and cheery, and never complain of aches and pains but are full of the sheer joy of living, one begins to get a glimpse of what is possible for each human being. One can also imagine this pristine health available to our ancestors, right into old age. Health is the "buoyancy of life, the infectious enthusiasm, the joy and insatiableness of play, the exuberance of energy and the ecstasy of living." (Shelton, *Health Review,* 1979, p. 1)

There are many people today who are very sick, and others who are borderline sick, and some who are apparently healthy, but we want everyone to experience exuberant health and be productive and creative human beings. Here is an invitation for everyone to experience perfect health.

Have you any conception of what "perfect health" means?

Can you form any image of how you would feel if every organ in your body were functioning perfectly? Perhaps you can go back to some day in your youth when you got up early in the morning and went for a walk: the spirit of the sunrise got into your blood, you walked faster, took deep breaths and laughed aloud for the sheer happiness of being alive in such a world of beauty. And now you have grown older – and what would you give for the secret of that glorious feeling? What would you say if you were told that you could bring it back and keep it, not only for mornings, but also for afternoons and evenings, and not as something accidental and mysterious, but also as something that you yourself have created and of which you are completely the master?

This invitation to health creates a new world, one where the individual begins to see oneself in a new way.

Everyone in the universe is seen differently. Nature and life become more beautiful and glorious.

"Duties which were irksome become easy to perform. We breathe purer atmosphere; new purposes animate us; new strength, energy and power are infused into us ... We see in every tree and shrub and every blade of grass a beauty of which we had not seen ... Our whole life is permeated by a spirit of love and goodwill; we develop a gentleness and kindness that is new to us. A fresh zeal enters into our relations ... strength is given ... with cheerfulness and delight. Troubles, anxieties and cares are dissipated." (Shelton, *Journal*, 1991, p.1)

HEALTH AS A NATURAL CONDITION

Good health is the normal state of the body. Children born of healthy parents are healthy at birth, and if given the proper care as infants, by being nursed and loved, remain healthy through childhood, growing into healthy adults to enjoy a productive long life. The children are disciplined easily, and are bright and co-operative. This is the natural state in humans as well as in animals.

The deterioration of health among children, adults and the elderly is an indication of the lack of knowledge available universally. By living according to the natural laws of life, these individuals can experience healthy bodies, sound minds and life to the fullest.

Good health is the birthright of every individual, providing they have the knowledge, will power and desire to stay well. "Prevention is better than cure" is an old proverb that teaches that health is experienced when remedial steps are taken to provide the body with its basic requirements for wellness, and to eliminate all harmful influences.

The body does not have to be made healthy: it is only necessary to provide the conditions for health and remove the cause of disease. In this way, one prevents interference with the body's healing power.

CONDITIONS NECESSARY FOR HEALTH

In health and disease it is of utmost importance to look at supplying the body with its basic needs so that it may build health, by removing all harmful influences that cause illness. The integrity of the organism strives towards health. The body in its wisdom heals itself.

The organism's vital action nourishes and develops organs, tissues, cells and body structures. This vital action, also known in Chinese philosophy as "Ch'i," or also known as nerve force, helps convert all elements of nutrition into body tissue and eliminates waste products as rapidly as they are created.

In investigating the factors in everyday life that could cause sickness, factors that can be derived from all aspects of the human personality – physical, mental, emotional or spiritual – then one can look at the whole person. Healing occurs when one can provide the conditions and circumstances necessary for health, providing the organism has not been irreversibly damaged in any way, in which case there would be limitations to regenerative progress. This would be found in those with degenerative diseases where there is the point of no return.

The restoration of health is not achieved by poisonous drugs, vaccines, surgery, or interference of any kind, but by supplying all the physiological needs of the body. With the body's capacity to use them at the time, and the removal of all the harmful effects of the illness, superior health will evolve,

Health is a gift and a virtue and it is available to everyone who seeks it. The symptoms one experiences in the body are a friendly signal that tells each individual that the laws of nature have not been followed. Obey the signal by adopting a healthy lifestyle.

This entails wholesome nutrition, mental and physical activity rest, sleep, emotional poise, pure water, fresh air, forgiveness, fasting to cleanse the body of stored excrement, and love of self and others. All this will create a productive life and will prevent the possibility of a life-threatening disease and ensure getting the only real security, that is, physical, mental and spiritual well-being for the rest of life.

To understand well-being one needs to look at the environment that supports it, and this means a change, sometimes a radical change, in the environment. This might mean getting a person out of their job, out of their city or out of any pressures in their existence in order to get well.

The rules of health have been made for the universe by the creator and have been scientifically proven over and over again. These laws of nature are based on fundamental biological principles. True health begins in the mind with understanding inner feelings.

Everything in the normal organism works towards optimum health. Each individual who wants to experience wellness is required to experience a supervised fast for quick effective results.

> "I have made a most exhaustive study of every method of cure from mind cure to modern surgery and gland therapy, and I have never found a single method that could approach even closely, in its results, the benefits which come from some form of fasting cure." (Dr. Frank McCoy, *The Fast Way to Health*, McCoy Publications, Inc., 1926, p. 17)

As an indulgent society, it becomes important to look at keeping well by knowing what constitutes health. Dr. Herbert Shelton describes it:

> "Health is the supreme virtue and it cannot be experienced

by one addicted to disease-producing habits. Reform means giving up habits that build disease and produce premature death. It means cultivating habits that build health and prolong life. (Dr. Herbert Shelton "Getting Well," *Health Research*, Mokalumne Hill, CA. p. 53)

In order for health to be experienced as widely as disease is prevalent today, teachers are needed who will emphasize the notion that when the cause of disease is removed, nature restores health and nature removes the effect. If the cause is an accumulation of toxic waste in the body, then the scientific world is required to search the knowledge available, as well as the therapeutic value of the oldest method of healing for the body, mind and soul, which is water fasting.

The best means of attaining and maintaining health are based in simple basic standards:

1. Cultivate emotional poise. Avoid worry, fear, anxiety, anger, self-pity, and jealousy and control the temper and passions.

2. Exercise daily, in the fresh air and sunshine is essential to physical and mental health. We are born to move. All the muscles in the body need exercise. Prevent weak bones by exercising. Vigorous exercise, but not to the point of fatigue, is best for good circulation.

3. Sleep comes easily to those who avoid stimulants. Rest in the afternoon if possible. The body regenerates during sound sleep and rest.

4. Secure enough sunshine every day; sunbathing in the nude is best. If this is not possible, then exposing the eyes and face to the sun helps to

metabolize calcium. The sun is an important nutritive raising the spirit, relieving depression and providing Vitamin D. Besides, the sun aids digestion and assimilation. Do not use sunscreens, lotions, sunglasses, or eyeglasses for best results.

5. Internal and external cleanliness, means the body, mind and especially the colon are to be kept clean. Bathing in clean water, and drinking pure water to keep the body clean is important. Fasting on water keeps the entire body clean by eliminating stored toxins.

6. Keep clean clothes, beds and homes.

7. Breathe fresh air. Keep windows open while sleeping. Get out of doors as often as possible.

8. Eat moderately of wholesome foods. Wholesome are fresh foods, unadulterated, not processed. Refined, manufactured, pickled, canned, preserved, cooked, etc.—all of these kinds of foods are deprived of mineral elements and vitamins and are usually bleached, colored, seasoned and preserved, all of which are unwholesome.

9. Clothing should be made of natural fabrics, i.e. cotton, wool, linen. And no tight bands, belts should be allowed to interfere with circulation.

10. Use the inherent talents to have an interest in life. A purposeful life is a rewarding and fulfilled life.

11. Avoid all Poison Habits: coffee, tea, cocoa, chocolate, tobacco, alcohol, opium, heroin, marijuana, soda fountain slops and other drugs, including sugar and salt. These all weaken, poison, and destroy the body.

12. Avoid all Excesses: Life depends on the conservation of energy. Be moderate and temperate in all things. Wasting energy by being over- indulgent impairs important bodily functions and builds toxins in the body destroying proper assimilation of foods and elimination of toxins.

13. Life is a struggle between self-control, which brings strength and happiness, and self-indulgence, which leads to misery and destruction.

14. Water is essential for cleansing the body and maintaining electrolyte balance, especially during a fast. There is no set rule as to how much water one requires, as it depends on a variety of factors, such as, activity, age, temperature, and the various foods eaten. If one eats concentrated food, flesh, salt, spices, sugar and processed foods, more water is required. If it is hot and one sweats, more water is needed. The best rules for drinking are: Drink fifteen minutes before meals or three hours after meals. It is best not to drink with meals as water and fluids taken with meals dilute the digestive juices and retards digestion.

NATURE'S LAWS FOR HEALTH

"....he who has health has hope
and he who has hope has everything"
– Arabian Proverb

The pain, suffering and premature death of many today are the direct and legitimate results of the violation of natural physical law. Obedience of the laws upon which life and health depend is the clue to health and lo t's ngevity.

As has been said by Harriet N. Austin, M.D.: "The first thing to be done is to teach the people that their life and health are put in their own keeping – and that sickness never comes without a cause, but is always the consequence of violation of the laws which regulate the human constitution." (*Health Science*, Austin's article, Nov. 1986, p. 106)

Accumulation of impurities from air, food, stress, drugs and other chemicals one ingests is a big cause of concern. Things that can cause sickness include:

- Deficient food created with modern technology, such as irradiation and genetic modification techniques
- Pesticides and fungicides in fruits and vegetables, whole grains, and nuts and seeds
- Addictive, heavily salted and spiced processed and deli foods
- Impure water

Several other factors can have a negative effect on health, creating a poor self-image affecting our intimate relations:

- Inadequate clothing and uncomfortable dwellings
- Overwork
- Inadequate sleep and rest
- Poor relationships with self and others
- Negative attitude, lack of forgiveness, and poor self-esteem

Every instance of sickness and suffering, unless caused by accident, is caused by wrongdoing.

Nature provides us with the following essential ingredients for health: Exercise daily, work that one loves, pure air, sunlight, whole foods, rest, sleep, emotional poise, pure water, positive attitude, and a great love for self, others and the universe.

Nature is a teacher and her warnings must be observed if health and long life are desired. Herbert Ratner, M.D. wrote, "Mother

Nature is a stern teacher ... who expects us to heed."

Health is a science based upon scientific facts dictated by natural laws as they apply to the human species. The human organism requires physiological and biological needs to maintain and restore health. When these needs are supplied, and the cause of disease is removed, then the living organism is self-sufficient, self-governing and can thrive in perfect health for the rest of life. If the organism is sick, then the conditions for health are applied and health returns.

From conception, human beings are endowed with a built-in program for a complete and fruitful life. Living organisms are self-programmed to meet all of life's needs within the environments of their adaptation.

The living organism is self-healing, provided the laws of nature are followed. The power that created life heals, and the power that repairs is the power that produces.

> "The power that evolves a full-grown individual from a fertilized ovum is the only healing power ... Healing is an intrinsic, not extrinsic power." (Shelton, *The Journal*, Nov. 1995, p. 2)

Health is a choice. The laws of life never change; they are eternal. The laws of nature never change; they are as sure as any laws of the universe. Once the human organism follows and knows the conditions for health and removes all the causes of disease, health is maintained and restored.

THE TRUE ESSENCE OF HEALTH

Health is wholeness. Co-operation with the immutable laws of nature will give humanity wellness and beauty, physically, mentally, emotionally and spiritually. All people have within a capability both to defend themselves against illness and to heal themselves when they become ill.

> "Nature – our subconscious – has a full monopoly on the power to cure. Healing is nature's prerogative, and she cannot, if she would, delegate it to doctors or the academies of medical science." (Dr. J.H. Tilden, M.D., 1960, p. 15)

The ability and strength to recognize nature's ways nurture all the basic needs of the organism. They are good, simple and provide health for a lifetime. The way we can recognize the signs of health is by knowing the qualities of health, as below.

1. Upon awakening there is no alarm clock and there is energy until the end of the day.

2. There is an urge to move upon awakening.

3. Healing occurs more quickly than anticipated. The faster the healing, the healthier one is.

4. There is a reflection of health when one looks in the mirror, with good posture and structure.

5. Flexibility and movement are natural and effortless.

6. Muscle strength is an indication of health.

7. There is stamina after suddenly having to run or jump.

8. There is an acute sense of sight, smell, hearing, taste and awareness.

9. The flesh is firm and solid, not flabby and wrinkled.

10. At the end of a day of hard work, sleep comes as soon as the head hits the pillow.

11. If feelings are hurt, i.e. after being rejected, jilted, ridiculed, etc., recovery comes easily and quickly and an optimistic attitude comes within a short time.

12. After making a mistake, forgiveness of self comes easily, as well as forgiveness towards others, soon after the incident occurs. To socialize and enjoy the company of others is appreciated.

13. One can stick to any current development in life that has been undertaken to enhance and expand abilities.

14. One experiences an adventurous spirit.

15. Anger is not expressed when annoyed or disturbed, nor is it bottled up inside. Expressing feelings is an important part of having good health.

16. Laughter and a smile happen often.

17. One accepts oneself and others unconditionally, with faults and virtues.

18. One experiences a positive, happy attitude towards life and has a great capacity for love and compassion for others.

HOW HEALTH IS DEPLETED

From conception, the organism is endowed with a built-in program for a full, complete and productive life. The human organism has two obligations to fulfill: to meet all of the biological rights and the environmental rights. The biological rights are: to breathe fresh air; to have sunlight; to eat wholesome, unadulterated foods; to have warmth and shelter, sleep, rest, recreation and work, that is, physical and mental activity; and the right to peace and tranquility. The environmental rights are:

each individual's right of privacy, ethics, code of conduct, the way one treats society and the way one treats the individual. The biological rights of each individual must be fulfilled and are most important. Health is achieved by healthful living. Biological and environmental rights not supplied for the human organism result in violence against the body, mind and spirit and against society.

Each individual is responsible for caring for the body. The graph indicates how health is destroyed.

HOW DISEASE IS BUILT
(as illustrated by the Tree of Bad Habits)

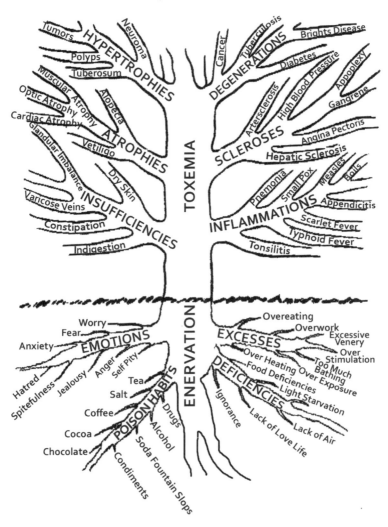

HEALTH IS A CHOICE

All healing power is inherent in the living organism. There is an order to life that has possessed the power to conceive, grow and develop. This same power is capable of healing its own ailments, repairing damages, protecting itself against injuries, preserving the integrity of its structures and enjoying longevity in a constructive, creative lifestyle.

> "It is vitality … vital force, nature, *vis medicatrix naturae*, etc. … that cures. That same force which brought us into being, which sustains us in existence, which has caused growth through all phases of life … enables one to move, act, think and is the power which must heal us…" (Dr. Walker, "Nutritive Cure," p. 16, *Health Science*, Mar. 1988)

Health is the product of living within natural law and order. A choice has to be made towards attaining health and the ideal society by living a normal healthy way of life in accordance with the laws of life. God, THE creator is the personification of all law and order. This is the power of intelligence and wisdom. To seek the knowledge of the structures and functions of the human body helps to establish the fact that health is the normal state of every human organism. Human beings are the most highly intelligent and organized in nature and can possess the highest degree of health. In the lower orders in nature, which have little intelligence and are simpler in construction, here superior health is found. It is in the lower order of nature that we see evidence of a low impairment and a greater observance to the laws of nature. For instance, one has to watch a cat that devours her meat and then lies down in a shady, quiet place to rest and recuperate. Upon waking she plays and romps, climbs, scratches and then finds a secluded spot to sun and sleep.

The level of health that individuals can attain will be in proportion to the degree they aspire to a state of perfectionism.

If led by health truths, health will expound and there will be no limits to it. To retrieve better health each human being must seek to discover the normal healthy way of life and discontinue all abuses and addictions. Education in right living has been neglected and the cause and remedy of all ailments needs to be resurrected in order that a choice can be made between health and disease.

> That "the average man is possessed of nothing more than the vaguest and generally incorrect views of the *modus operandi* of causes operating in the lives of people is not grounds for accepting … erroneous conclusions about the … the importance of a correct mode of living." (Shelton, *Health Review,* Nov. 1972, p. 255)

In a state of health there is sufficient nerve energy to sustain all the functions in the body adequately to meet the ordinary demands of life and still be able to leave a reserve supply for an emergency. Health rejects, from its *materia medica*, all poisons that are destructive to the living organism. Health is no accident, neither is disease, but is a direct result of living according to nature's laws. Each individual is responsible for the conditions of attaining and maintaining good health. Health is a decision and is innate in every living being. All individuals have to seek the truth about health by knowing all the prerequisites to health and by removing the causes of disease. Health is a responsible choice made by all who care about life.

WHAT TO EAT

In Genesis I: 29, when humans were first created, the Creator said, "Look, to you I give you all the seed bearing plants everywhere on the surface of the earth, and all the trees with seed bearing fruit, this will be your food"

It is interesting to note that when people are sick, in pain or diseased and they follow this plan, they all experience healing in a very short time.

Our daily choices of food manifest the harmony we have with ourselves, our relationships, with the world, creation, the earth and the Divine. Our food has a direct influence on the peace we create with ourselves and the whole world.

The human body does best with live, whole, fresh organic foods. The food most adaptable to the human physiology is a plant-based dietary plan of organically grown raw fresh fruits and vegetables, nuts and seeds and whole grains; the correct balance is eighty percent alkaline and twenty percent acid foods.

We must eat enough uncooked food to offset fermentation and to supply the vitamins and mineral salts necessary to build health and strength. If one chooses to eat some cooked food, it is necessary to eat the greater portion of food uncooked to supply the raw materials for the human body.

Sunflower

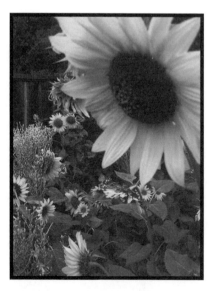

Vibrancy - Nourishment - Longevity

CHAPTER II

Much of your pain is self-chosen.
It is the bitter potion by which the physician within you
heals your sick self.
Therefore trust the physician,
and drink his remedy in silence and tranquility:
For his hand, though heavy and hard
is guided by the tender hand of the Unseen,
And the cup he brings, though it burn your lips,
has been fashioned of the clay
which the Potter has moistened
with His own sacred tears.
— *The Prophet*, Kahlil Gibran, p. 52-53

THE BASIC CAUSE OF DISEASE

There is an ancient theory that disease is an organized substance or force existing outside the body and that it is at war with life. It is a law of life that the body resists and expels whatever it cannot use. Therefore, disease is vital resistance to non-usable, injurious substances. The human organism grows and reproduces itself. The human body develops its parts and continually repairs itself by selecting such materials from its environment as it has the capacity to incorporate into its own structures, and rejects and refuses everything else as injurious.

"The power of refusal and rejection is a necessary condition of its vital integrity. Refusal and rejection are constant actions in both plants and animal world." (Shelton, *Health Review,* Mar. 1979, p. 251-54)

The difference between health and disease is that health is the normal performance of all functions of the body, or physiology. Disease is abnormal or irregular action of the body in expelling injurious substances and repairing damages; in other words, pathology. Health nourishes and develops the body, organs, tissues, cells, building unity, or the conversion of food into elements of body tissue, and the elimination of waste. In disease, poisons are eliminated and damages repaired. It is the action of the same powers that are present in health, in defending the body against injurious substances and conditions present in disease.

"The nature of disease is explained the same way that the modus operandi of drugs is explained. The immediate effect of the introduction of a drug, or poison, into the body is morbid vital action. This is disease. The action of the organism against any repugnant or poisonous substance is defensive – it is an effort to dispose of the offending material. Purging occasioned by a drug is a perfect illustration of diarrhea or dysentery. Vomiting from an emetic is carried on in the same way, and for the same purpose that vomiting from any other cause is carried on." (Shelton, *Health Review,* July 1973, p. 254)

The symptoms given by the body are messages and are evidences of vitality. Dead bodies do not produce symptoms.

"Deprive the living organism of its ability to manifest its repugnance to incompatible things, its power to reject and resist these, in the defensive manner, that we call disease, and you deprive it of life itself." (Shelton, *Health Review,* p. 254)

If the body has lost its vitality or nerve energy, which is necessary for recuperation, then the organism will not react powerfully to the abnormal condition of disease.

Symptoms are vital actions given by the vital organs of the body. Health is the regular or normal performance of all the functions and organs, tissues and cells of the body and this is called physiology. Disease is abnormal action of the body trying to expel injurious substances and repair damage, also called pathology. Disease is vital action of the body to remove anything harmful so that the body functions can be balanced. It is not evil and it is not so much an outside influence as much as it is an internal vital action taken by the body to correct itself.

THE UNITY OF HEALTH AND DISEASE

"No one can experience perfect health because health is an ongoing thing. Health is more than the absence of disease. People look at health and disease as antagonistic opposites, as though they are opposing forces. Health and disease are not static conditions, but both are fluctuating qualities of the living organism. Most individuals are sick, a little or a whole lot, and no one can claim to be one hundred percent healthy. It is everyone's birthright to be well all the time to a greater or lesser degree. Even the man who is dying is still experiencing a certain degree of health. " (Dr. Gerald Benesh's speech at a Natural Health Conference, Windsor, Ontario, July 1974)

"We think of health and disease as a continuum, with health at the top in the ideal position. As we go down the scale health becomes less and less, and of course, we get into disease." (Dr. Alec Burton, *Health Science*, Mar. 1980, p. 200)

To be at the top and have ideal health, a person would have to have had generations of healthful living. An individual may not be able to reach the ideal; however, improvement can be made.

All the necessary prerequisites for health are the same as those needed when in the state of disease. That is, fresh air, whole foods, pure water, emotional poise, mental and physical activity, cleanliness, both external and internal – as in fasting – rest, sleep and relaxation, moderate sunlight, and love for self and others.

All the harmful influences that negate health are the same as those that cause disease. These are: refined and processed foods with additives, preservatives, fungicides and pesticides; beverages of coffee, tea, chocolate and soft drinks, as well as other non-nutritious substances that individuals consume which introduce sources of toxins into the body; drugs and chemicals; stress and the lack of emotional poise that also contribute to the absorption of decomposing products within the organism.

In examining the way of life of the individual it is important to find out what is done or not done for the organism that could prevent wellness. The removal of the cause of disease is of utmost importance. To provide a program that will provide the conditions and circumstances necessary for health will restore the organism to balance. In chronic degenerative diseases that could have had some irreversible damages there could be some limitations as to regenerative processes.

The environment of the individual and how it supports the health of the organism is important. A change of the environment may be of great importance. For instance, it may mean a change of job, a change of location, ending a relationship, or whatever may be causing stress.

Disease Is Not an Enemy

Disease is a friendly message from the body that says there is something the body requires that might have been neglected, or there are harmful influences getting in the way of healing. Listen to the messages of the body, which will provide the security of ensuring physical and mental well-being. Symptoms are messages from the intelligent organism that is trying to remedy a problem and is striving to improve the internal environment. The individual who does not interfere with the remedial process of the body sees the reparative and defensive influences as the only method that heals. Illness is made up of symptom complexities and a cure for the symptom means to suppress the body's own remedial process.

The body produces toxins every day, and if it fails to excrete them adequately and quickly, then a crisis, such as a cold, fever, or flu, will develop. Also, nutritional inadequacies or oversupply stress the body and then one can see disease as a process of repair and regeneration.

> "Disease has no independent existence. Nobody has ever seen disease. For instance, diarrhea is one of the symptoms associated with some diseases." (Dr. Alec Burton's article in *Health Science*, Feb. 1980, p. 202)

As the body attempts to heal itself, human beings try to prevent this process by suppression.

In health and disease the main concern is to remove the cause of disease and to supply the organism with all the basic needs so it can attain and maintain health. Disease is created and health is the natural tendency toward the ideal.

Let education in health teach the individual to stop creating disease.

The laws of life are to be followed in order to experience health. The laws are based on fundamental biological principles. For instance, if a patient is under too much stress, the stress has to be eliminated; otherwise the individual continues to deteriorate.

The whole person and their way of life, such as the basic needs, feelings, attitudes and influences are to be studied. Health begins in the mind, and it is here that important decisions are made and health developed

Health is more than a feeling. It is physiological and biological and based upon these factors.

> "It is a state of wholeness – of structural integrity and functional efficiency – based on … living and wholesome biological relations." (Dr. Herbert Shelton, *Getting Well*, 1960, p. 14)

This means that biologically and physiologically the body performs efficiently and with integrity all the necessary functions of the body. This will happen only when all of the conditions of health are provided, and all harmful influences are removed and a new mode of life has begun.

Owl

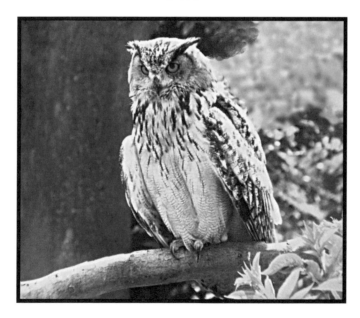

Intelligence – Wisdom – Brilliance – Intuition

CHAPTER III

Health is normal. Disease is abnormal.
*The Creator intended that every human being
should have health.
If we do not it means that we have
broken some of Nature's laws*

WHAT IS DISEASE

Disease in the body is a result of the body's inability to keep itself clear of its own accumulated debris. Disease is a remedial action. This means it is a process of purification and reparation. In an extract from a discourse delivered by Russell T. Trall, M.D., on the March 25, 1863, to the New York Senate, he clarifies the mystery of disease.

> "Disease is not a thing to be suppressed, subdued, broken up, destroyed, conquered, 'cured', or killed, but an action to be directed and regulated." (Shelton, *Health Review,* Nov. 1973, p. 58)

In disease, an effort is made by the body to cleanse the areas that are obstructed.

> "A special effort is made by the vital powers to cleanse the system to rid itself of the presence of infections,

poisons, or impurities. This special effort – a remedial action – is the disease." (Shelton, *Health Review*, Nov. 1973, p. 60)

As the vital organs try to expel the built-up waste, or remedial action, the brain is deprived of blood and nervous energy, causing disorder.

The term used in medical schools, *vis medicatrix naturae*, and disease, are not antagonistic principles but *vis medicatrix naturae* is disease and they are the same. This means that the life force that heals and gives health and disease, or discomfort, where the body is trying to restore itself to health, are not enemies at war, but "on the contrary both are the same vital powers in an effort to expel from the system injurious things and to repair the damages which their presence has occasioned." (Shelton, *Health Review*, Nov. 1973, p. 60)

The same system, the medical system, which aims to cure disease with potent medication, "can be nothing more or less than a war on the human constitution." (Shelton, p. 60) In other words, disease is abnormal action; health is normal action of the body's vital life force trying to keep everything functioning at its best. For instance health continually converts the elements of food into new cells, tissues and organs: disease is the action of the same vital force in defense of injurious substances or abnormal conditions, using its power to expel harmful substances.

> "Health and disease are, in the organic domain, precisely what peace and war are among nations. One is productive industry and the other is destructive, but leads to remedial action. Health is the *vis conservatrix naturae* and disease is the *vis medicatrix naturae*. One is order and the other disorder." (Shelton, p. 60)

Un-eliminated waste products is one of the primary causes of disease, illness, degeneration, premature old age, and suffering, as well as cruelty, crime, poor relationships, anger, hostility, a short fuse, and poor self-esteem. This vital action is designed to resist and expel poisons and to repair damages in the body. All disease and illness are cleansing efforts of the body.

> "It is one of the fundamental powers of biological forms to select, to choose, to reject … In resisting and expelling non-usable materials (poisons) the body acts defensively. It seeks to preserve itself from harm." (Shelton, *Health Review*, Dec. 1973, p. 252)

The human organism selects those raw materials that will nourish and sustain health, and that which it cannot use it resists. This occurs when the individual is healthy and the symptoms experienced are evidences of vitality. There are two sets of processes alive in a vital body: one, the body transforms the raw materials into tissue, organs, and cells, and throws off unused waste matter; this is called health. The other process expels foreign or injurious substances and repairs damages; this is called disease.

The *vis medicatrix naturae*, which is the body's vital struggle in self-defense, or the process of purification, is called the disease itself.

> "So far from the disease and the *vis medicatrix naturae* being antagonistic entities or forces at war with each other, they are one and the same" (Russell Trall, M.D. *The True Healing Art*, 1970, p. 91)

Disease, or the lack of ease, in ancient times, as well as today, is considered to be an attack upon the human organism by an outside force or entity. For instance, a fever is caused by the same powers of life that produce normal body temperature. All physiological actions, or vital actions by the body, normal or abnormal, as Dr. Shelton describes, "are caused by the same vital or physiological powers. Outside forces do not cause the actions of the body. The cause of vital actions is resident in the living organism." (Shelton, *Getting Well*, p. 17)

The "vital actions" are the defensive action, or the recuperative actions of the body, and these are called disease. Also, the condition of injury, cut, etc., produced by poisons, fire, toxins, etc., is called disease. There have been many discoveries for the cure of disease and preventives, such as vaccines and serums; and today more research is done to find that universal health answer to combat disease, yet needless suffering continues.

In the search for cures and prevention one has to ask: Are the medical establishments suppressing symptoms, or removing the cause of disease? If the cause of disease is not removed, then a cure will not happen. For instance, does surgery remove the cause of the illness? True health conquers disease as it meets all the normal biological means of life and avoids the harmful influences. Fresh air, pure water, whole foods, grown on balanced soil, sunlight, rest, sleep, mental and physical activity, fasting, or having a physiological rest, and loving self and others, are the basic needs of the body.

Avoid salt, sugar, coffee tea, alcohol, tobacco, drugs, preservatives and additives in foods, since all are harmful to the sensitive organism and all cause illness.

For instance, salt is un-assimilable as it is a crude, inorganic substance which is absorbed by the intestine unchanged, causing retention, irritating delicate mucous membranes and disturbing fluid balances and electrical balance of nerve cells, causing degeneration and organ dysfunction, such as arthritis, cancer, etc.

Salt retards digestion and retards the ability to absorb vitamins, changes blood chemistry, paralyzes the inner lining of the blood vessels, stimulates the heart, retards kidney function and paralyzes the secretory activities. Salt causes excess weight gain and increases the appetite. (Weight Loss Diet Book, p. 49) It is unwholesome and un-nutritious, and the human organism cannot metabolize it.

Sodium is necessary, not sodium chloride as this is a poison to the body.

Health is built upon these simple natural laws. This is the valid means of restoring and preserving health. At this time one can say a move has been made from cure to CARE.

The human body is created in this way because nature needs no cure; it heals itself if all the necessary prerequisites of the body are met and the harmful influences eliminated.

DISEASE AS A REMEDIAL PROCESS

Fever, being one of the simplest remedial actions of the body trying to burn off poisons, is a process of purification. "A fever must be one of the methods in which the system relieves itself of morbid matter." (Russell Trall, M.D., *The True Healing Art,* 1970, p. 95)

There is profound simplicity in understanding disease when one can see it as a vital action taken by the body to restore itself to normalcy through eliminating stored waste materials. Illness is the vital struggle of the body in self-defense. If poisons cause disease, then how do these non-usable materials get saturated in the blood, lymph, tissues and cells?

ENERVATION

The first stage in the diversion of the human body from normal health is the use of more nerve energy than is normally produced. This expenditure of more energy than rest and sleep can restore is called enervation. In violating the laws of life, the powers of healing that normally heal become feeble and deprive the body of its excretory functions; as well the assimilative powers become weakened, causing inadequate nourishment. In order for the body to be able to restore itself back to normal, sufficient rest, sleep and pure water is necessary so that the body can eliminate stored toxins. This stored waste accumulates and the individual may experience abnormal mucous secretions or discharges. This is the beginning of a pathological condition. The depletion of nerve energy creates toxemia because of the imperfect elimination and the lack of good assimilation of nutrients. Toxemia builds disease.

TOXEMIA

The blood and lymphatic systems become foul and no longer protect the body. General or constitutional toxemia exists long before the so-called local disease develops and without the constitutional toxemia, there would be no "local disease."

> "Fermentation and putrefaction are common all-around influences ... pathological fermentation is sure to occur, not because of the presence of germs ... but because of abnormal secretions which do not protect from fermentation. This gives rise to poisons which are absorbed causing infection." (Shelton, *Health Review*, March 1973, p.155)

There are two sources of toxemia, poisons or impurities taken into the organism from without, and waste matter retained. The result is obstruction, or the cause of disease. The vital effort of the body to remove the obstructing material from the body and repair damages is the beginning of healing. This is remedial action.

> "It is a vital struggle to overcome obstructions and to keep the channels of the circulation free and should this self-defensive action, this remedial effort, this purifying process,

this attempt at reparation, this war for the integrity of the living organism, this contest against the enemies of the organic constitution, repressed by bleeding, or suppressed with drugs, intensified with stimulants and tonics, subdued with narcotics and antiphlogistics, confused with blisters and caustics, aggravated with alteratives, and confused and misdirected, changed, subverted and perverted with drugs and poisons generally... To give drugs is adding to the causes of disease, for drugs always produce disease." (Russell Trall, *The True Art of Healing*, 1970, p. 44)

James C. Jackson, M.D., who contributed much to prevention and the care of the patient in his book written in 1860, in an article on "The Gluttony Plague," says this about habits:

"We pay high prices for a method of introducing deadly poison into our life-currents easier by far than that which vaccination offers. (Jackson, p. 89) And, "The great indifference to the Laws of Life ... the impunity with which they are violated ... the laws of health are absolutely essential for the maintenance of normal function, but when normal activity has been established, or recovery occurs, there are certain conditions that a human being must meet as a social being." (Jackson, p. 88)

In pronounced toxemia, any irritated mucous membrane will be required to do vicarious eliminative work. Where habits cause impairment, the departure from the normal is a pathological change with the weakest organ offering the least resistance to the toxins.

"Toxemia is the presence in the blood, lymph, secretions and cells, of any substances, from any source, which, in sufficient quantity, will impair organic functions. Toxemia means the presence of too great a percentage of toxins in the tissues and fluids of the body." (Herbert M. Shelton, *Health For All*, p. 19)

Due to continuous enervating habits, the next stage of pathology develops: irritation, such as sinusitis, ulceration, or chronically inflamed tissue, which evolves into induration or hardening, which has three endings, those being fungation or cancer, tuberculosis and other degenerative diseases. All these crises pass when the toxins have been reduced to the toleration point. All enervating habits must be eliminated in order for health to return, and a healthy lifestyle and attitude taken seriously. Harriet N. Austin, M.D., wrote,

> "Sickness is always caused by wrong doing. The first thing to be done is to teach the people that their life and health are put into their own keeping, and that sickness never comes without a cause, but is always the consequences of violation of the laws which regulate the human constitution." (*Eternal Health Truths*, p. 106)

To suppress disease has not taught the patient what caused it. As Dr. Shelton states,

> "To subdue or 'regulate' these expressions is to thwart nature's efforts at eliminating the causes of damaged structure and restoring health. Such measures can never restore health, although the body is often able to restore health in spite of them." (Shelton, *Getting Well*, p. 66)

Symptoms teach individuals that change is necessary. Change means the removal of the cause of illness so that the organism can be restored to normal.

BUILDING A STRONG IMMUNE SYSTEM

The T-cells, which mature in the thymus gland, are the internal monitors of our immune system. The B-cells produced by bone marrow patrol the organism for invaders.

A constant movement occurs between the invaders and the

monitoring system. Stress sabotages this defense system and creates enervation and toxemia. Certain foods and beverages do the same. Stressors on the emotional level are grief, job loss, social problems, infections, excessive fatigue, exposure to heat or cold, medication, operations or the death of a loved one.

The foods that sabotage the immune system are: caffeine, pop, drugs, coffee, and tea; because of their diuretic properties, potassium and other minerals are lost from the body. A potassium deficiency can lead to an irregular heartbeat. Caffeine being a deadly poison creates stress for the nervous system and heart and is a strain on the body by having to metabolize a deadly acid-forming substance, depositing insoluble cellulose in the liver. Caffeine is also heavy in pesticides.

Chocolate contains theobromide, a stimulant similar to caffeine; Phenylethylamine, an amphetmine-like chemical; also traces of compounds similar to tetrahydrocannabinol or THC, the active ingredient in marijuana. These are all traces of mild opiates, which target the same part of the brain as heroin or morphine, thus addictive, creating a feeling of well-being. Although organic chocolate is available and is heavily advertised as being high in antioxidants, it is not recommended on a health supporting diet. Also chocolate contains refined sugar, and oxalic acid, which prevents the body from metabolizing calcium.

Sugar, white flour, salt, white rice, and fragmentations of food rob the body of iron, calcium and other nutrients.

Animal products, particularly high in protein and saturated fats, cause putrefaction in the intestinal tract and are also known to cause cancer, heart disease and degenerative diseases.

Dr. Neal Barnard, M.D., founder and president of the Physicians Committee for Responsible Medicine, and editor of "Good Medicine" in Washington, D.C., says,

"It's no big surprise that vegetarians have much less risk of heart disease, cancer, diabetes, hypertension, kidney problems, and even appendicitis, compared to meat-eaters."(*Good Medicine*, Vol. X, No. 3, Summer 2001)

Condiments (spices, vinegar) contain acetic acid, which is highly toxic, and destroys ptyalin, the salivary enzyme necessary to converts starch into sugar. In the book, *The Original Natural Hygiene Weight Loss Diet Book*, written by Dr. H. Shelton, Jean Oswald and Jean Oswald, they say:

"Experiments have shown that a small portion of vinegar as one in 5,000 appreciably diminishes the digestion of starch." (p.48) It also contains alcohol, which precipitates the pepsin of the gastric juice and prevents gastric digestion of proteins, and this includes apple cider vinegar. Thus digestion is impaired in using anything containing vinegar.

Fried foods are responsible for skin cancer, heart disease, and high blood pressure, because they cause free radicals, which are unstable molecules that deplete the immune system and are precursors of cancer. Tobacco is a strong pollutant of our blood stream.

HOW TO PROTECT THE IMMUNE SYSTEM

Be content with loving the work one does. Know how to relax under pressure and have a good relationship with self and others. Learn to let go, love and forgive. At the same time, provide the organism with all of the necessary prerequisites for health.

SUPPRESSION OF DISEASE

Those treated for colds, influenza and viruses have a longer period of disability than those untreated, prolonging the disease as well as increasing the possibility that the acute problem will develop into a chronic disease or other disability. Dr. O.P.J. Falk, M.D., Assistant Professor of Clinical Medicine, St. Louis University School of Medicine, said this about cures:

> "In virus infections such as colds and influenza, the diaphoretic drugs (those that increase perspiration) such as aspirin and phenacetin, appear to make the individual more susceptible to complicating superimposed bacterial infections and perhaps favor extension of the original virus involvement."

Falk also says that in reducing fever artificially, there are physiologic disadvantages.

> "We have contended that in thus suppressing symptoms, the medical man prolongs the patient's illness, converts acute into chronic disease and kills the patient ... and suppressive treatment is the chief cause of 'complications.'" (Shelton, *Health Review*, Dec. 1972, p. 91-92) Dr. Shelton continues to note: "Medicine as it is taught and practiced today, is a system of spectacular palliation. Falk continues to argue the effects of drugs, 'It is known ... that penicillin or the newer mycin types of antibiotics have no specific effect on virus infections. Antibiotics do not tend to prevent super-imposed complicating bacterial infections, when used in the early stages of an acute infection, as has been claimed by some physicians.'"

In every disease it is found that the effects of drugs create a negative and more serious condition. "The evil effects of drugs are often much worse than those produced by the cause of arthritis." In this case, arthritis treated as an infection by a living agent.

> "To suppress symptoms leads to a more complicated disease. Like the aspirin and phenacetin, which appear

to make the individual 'more susceptible' to colds, these anti-arthritis drugs render the arthritis worse." (Shelton, *Health Review*, Dec. 1972, p. 92)

The more healthy the individual, the more violent will be the reaction of the body towards eliminating any foreign substance in order to house-clean. The human body in the state of good health is a

"virile, dynamic structure that may be as violent in its voluntary actions as it often is in its voluntary activities. When the occasion calls for violence, it acts with great violence ... the violent actions of the body have been mistaken for something else – of disease, poisons, etc." Yet, it is the organism's intelligence to create homeostasis and be well again. (Shelton, *Health Review*, Aug. 1972, p. 279)

It may appear complicated that the healthy reactions of the body to expel a substance, such as in diarrhea or vomiting, constitute what is called disease. Sylvester Graham pioneered health programs in the 1830s and wrote and lectured on the Science of Human Life that,

"the stronger and more healthy an organism is, the more prompt and violent will be its actions in expelling a poison; the weaker and less virile the organism the slower and less vigorous will be its defensive and reparative activities." (Sylvester Graham, M.D., *Lectures on the Science of Human Life*, 1883, Fowler & Wells, Publishers, p. 828)

Colds, fevers, vomiting, nausea, diarrhea, etc., are what Dr. Russell Trall called "life preserving actions." Dr. Trall defines disease as "remedial action." Disease is not merely abnormal action; it is action with a purpose. It is designed to resist and expel poisons to repair damage. (Shelton, *Health Review*, Aug. 1972, p. 280) The simple cold and the rash are indications that a poison has gathered slowly and the tissues are overloaded with waste and the body in self-defense is trying to expel the excess material. These are all indications of the powerful healing and cleansing efforts of the body. It is at this time that the human organism requires rest – a physiological rest – a fast, in order to rapidly clean and restore itself to health.

In a study lesson on "Poisoning the Sick," Dr. Herbert Shelton stated,

> "It is the general opinion that people die of disease and that they are sometimes prevented from dying by taking poisons." (Shelton, *The Educator*, Aug. 1974, p. 3) Shelton also says, "Poison is always a destroyer of living organisms, while there is ample evidence to show that disease is constructive effort on the part of the body to rid itself of poisons … people die of poisoning, violence and exhaustion."

Dr. Russell Trall questions remedies for the sick:

> "When these remedies are given to well persons they produce, more or less, nausea, vomiting, purging, pain, heat, swelling, gripping, vertigo, spasms, stupor, coma, delirium, and death. When they are given to sick persons they produce the same manifestations of disease, modified by the condition of the patient and the circumstances of the prior disease." (Shelton, *Health Review*, Aug. 1974, p. 28l)

Drugs are poisons that affect the tissues and structures of the body and create complications harmful to the human organism. Dr. Shelton further informs:

> "To say that certain 'remedies' kill germs, viruses, parasites, is to overlook the fact that they also kill the cells of the body, and often the whole body."

Dr. Shelton also illustrates that when Dr. Walter was given medicine by a physician and placed the vial containing the drug in his vest pocket, he says, "the cork came out and the liquid contents soaked my clothing, it ate away part of the vest, burned holes in the shirt and I mourned over the loss of what evidently had 'strength' in it as he was supposed to take the drug internally."

Research is conducted on drugs for a multitude of diseases. This is costly and patients do not learn the cause of the illness by masking the symptoms with a remedy. Dr. Shelton says,

> "It is a strange practice that a remedy which always tends to kill is always chosen to cure the sick ... The physician is a product of education ... We have defined a poison as a substance which is not, in any quantity, convertible into any of the structures and substances of the living body and is not employed by the organism in the performance of any of its functions." (Shelton, *Health Review*, Aug. 1974, p. 2)

The human organism is self-repairing. Poisons given to a patient do not remove the cause of the illness. Poisons are chemically incompatible with the functions of human life. Dr. Trall said this at the Smithsonian Institution:

> "Drug medication, no matter in what disguise nor under what name it is practiced, consists in employing, as remedies for disease, those things which produce disease in well persons. Its *materia medica* is simply a list of drugs, chemicals in a word, poisons." (Shelton, *Health Review*, Aug. 1974, p. 2)

To care for the sick and to prevent illness means to remove the cause of disease and preserve health by supplying all the conditions for health.

GERMS DO NOT CAUSE DISEASE

Germs are present in disease but do not cause it. Germs are very toxic when in excess as they live off dead and decayed matter. Bacteria are necessary for normal body functions as they decompose excretions and help in the elimination. When the body secretions and excretions are normal, bacteria are harmless. When toxemia exists, that is having more toxic material than the body can eliminate, then the accumulated waste material create abnormal and poisonous substances that are harmful to the body. Dr. Shelton states,

> "Bacteria excrete toxic waste only when human secretions are abnormal and when cells of the body are in a low state of vitality. When many cells of the body are killed by excessive toxic saturation, bacteria go to work to disorganize them and help the body rid itself of dead tissue." (Shelton, *Health Review*, May 1975, p. 5)

It is important to keep the environment of the organism healthy and clean to prevent excess bacteria from creating a heavy toxic load in the body. If the environment is toxic, the bacteria will become virulent. If the environment of the body is clean, then the bacteria will be normal for healthy function of the whole organism.

THE CAUSE OF TOXEMIA

The environment in which one lives creates an unnatural condition for self-renewing and self-repairing of organs, tissues and cells. The body is created to last well over a hundred years. It is our excesses, deficiencies and stress that are the major contributions towards illness. As one looks at the food most human beings consume, it is food grown on deficient soil. Food derived from soil that is inadequate, or where fungicides and pesticides are used in the growing, will also be lacking in the essential vitamins and minerals. The human diet is composed of natural, organic whole foods; that is, fresh fruit and vegetables, nuts and seeds and whole grains. The food consumed daily needs to be wholesome, and as close to its natural state as possible. This will have a bearing on preserving health and the prevention of disease.

Denatured foods will not digest properly because of their lack of enzymes. These foods will not nourish the body completely. Dr. Virginia Vetrano, assistant to Dr. Herbert Shelton for many years, says,

> "See that your food is natural and wholesome and you will have taken a big step toward preventing enervation and the development of disease." (Shelton, *Health Review*, May 1975, p. 10)

Exercise also prevents toxemia. The body becomes strong with regular exercise. Dr. Vetrano says, "It is necessary for strength, vitality and mind development." Endurance increases and digestive capacities are improved with regular activity. Elimination is improved and decomposition of food is less likely to occur when exercise is taken seriously.

Sunlight is important for normal functioning of the body. Vitamin D is important to health and without sunlight it cannot be assimilated. This will prevent calcium from being manufactured in the body. The sun shining upon the skin produces Vitamin D. Dr. Vetrano states,

> "It has been shown that light picked up by the retina and passing by way of optic nerve influences the body by nerve impulses reaching the endocrine system. All bodily functions can be influenced by sunshine and light." (Shelton, *Health Review*, May 1975)

Sleep deprivation will have a negative effect on bodily functions. Rest is essential for repair and rejuvenation of the body. Sleep and rest restore nerve energy. The final consequence of lack of rest is that toxemia builds up, and disease takes over. The accumulation of metabolic waste materials is excessive and the body becomes fatigued and deprived of nourishment.

Enervation and toxemia do not develop in the organism that supplies the conditions for health and eliminates all harmful influences. Dr. Vetrano also says in the same article,

> "To maintain superb health from infancy to old age, we must learn what causes disease and avoid the cause … we must prevent enervation by supplying all deficiencies of things normal to physiology, and by not going to excess in any of the things normal to physiology, by avoiding all poison habits, and learning to control our emotions." (Shelton, *Health Review*, May 1975)

IMMUNIZATION

The cause of disease is not because of bacteria; therefore, it is unnecessary to inject antibodies into the bloodstream. A healthy body forms antibodies. The human body's own antibodies and white blood cells can destroy bacteria, foreign substances and toxic material. Foreign antibodies are rejected by the body as foreign protein and are not used but only help to poison the body and lower the immune system. Antibodies are formed by a healthy body to destroy bacteria and poisons that enter into the system.

The human organism has a natural resistance against all foreign substances. The body considers foreign proteins found in vaccines a poison and tries to expel it. Dr. Herbert Shelton states,

> "The injected foreign antibody becomes an antigen, i.e. that which is capable of causing an immune response in the body. This means that the body has to produce antibodies against a foreign antibody, which is in reality

an antigen. An antigen is a substance causing the body to produce antibodies against it, to help eliminate it from the system." (Shelton, *Health Review*, May 1975)

An extra expenditure of nerve energy is required in order to eliminate this foreign substance. The body becomes enervated and more toxemia develops. Immunization creates enervation, toxemia, and a body more susceptible to disease.

The body has to eliminate a poison because it cannot be utilized. Vital structure can be obtained out of wholesome food, pure water, sunshine, exercise, emotional poise, rest and sleep. If the body cannot assimilate it then it is a poison and, therefore, the body tries to reject it by expelling it. Dr. Shelton states,

> "Many drugs produce no appreciable immediate damage but are retained, as they are eliminated with difficulty, and accumulate in the body and it is said by toxicologists of some of these that small amounts of such drugs may be retained in the body for months and even years." (Shelton, *Man's Pristine Way of Life*, 1968, p. 466)

If not eliminated, drugs produce disease when in contact with the tissues of the organism. It is safe to say and has been proven scientifically, that those vaccinated have often contracted the disease for which they were inoculated. Dr. Shelton goes on to say, "Vaccination is a dangerous, a damaging and damnable fraud and only the most ignorant and superstitious can believe in it." (Shelton, *Health Review*, Oct. 1991, p. 19)

Vaccinations do not protect one against disease, but they impair health. Prevention of disease requires that each individual stop doing what is harmful to the organism and pro vide the body with the conditions for health.

VIRUSES AND DISEASE

Viruses are found only in late stages of disease processes, in decomposing dead cells and waste products, which explains that the virus is a by-product of disease, not the cause of it.

The word "virus" has a double meaning: It means poison, or the toxic products of decomposing organic wastes. Joklik & Willettt in *Zinsser Microbiology*, 16th edition, state,

> "The foot-and-mouth disease produced by Loeffler and Frosch was also a case of poisoning from the wastes of toxemic cattle; Sir Albert Howard observed, when he was raising cattle upon organically grown feeds and composted pasture, that when his cows touched the cows with foot-and-mouth disease from an adjoining farm through the fence, his did not get the disease." (p. 70)

The neighboring cows got the disease because they were fed from depleted soil and were malnourished. By improving the feed, the cows with the disease recovered quickly. Malnourishment was the cause of disease, not the virus. Virus is also known as "a nucleic acid fragment with protein coating," says Dr. Alec Burton in an article entitled, "What is a virus." These fragments are found in dead cells as they decompose, and they join with the genetic material of bacteria. (*The Journal*, Oct. 1995, p. 9)

Viruses and bacteria are part of the ecosystem, a part of nature; they do not cause disease. They are the result of excess waste material accumulated in the organism, as a result of the manner in which one lives.

Dr. Burton, in one of his lectures at a health conference, defines health as living symptom-free. The healthy person has a balance of viruses and bacteria, or germs. He also added, "virus is not the cause of Aids; rather it is caused by the environment, by sexual practices, by a lack of attention to diet, rest, exercise, stress and many other factors." (Dr. Burton's Lecture, Health Conference, Windsor, Ontario, Canada, July 1972)

It is the habits that lead one to disease. Drugs depress the immune system and damage the organism. The cure for viruses has nothing to do with the cause of the disease they are meant to cure. Living in accordance with the natural God-given laws that govern the human body prevents serious viruses and disease.

Acute, chronic and degenerative diseases are the organism's attempt to purify itself and get back to homeostasis. Dr. Emmet Densmore, M.D., in 1891 wrote: "Disease is actually a friendly expression on the part of the system of an effort to rid itself of conditions and substances inimical to health." (*How Nature Cures*, p. 56)

Dr. John H. Tilden, M.D., who wrote *Toxemia, The Basic Cause of all Disease* after fifty years of active medical practice, said, "An acute affection (disease) is simply an effort on the part of the body to right itself, and if left to itself it will succeed; but among civilized people Nature is recognized as a fool, and every effort that she makes to right herself is met by the opposition of so-called scientific medicine, and her efforts are suppressed." (*Toxemia Explained*, 1960, p. 58; also found in *Criticisms of the Practice of Medicine*, 1909, p. 198)

The symptoms of these diseases are not the disease; they are the consequences of the disease or imbalance, and the organism's attempt to heal itself.

THE BODY HEALS ITSELF

To remove the cause of disease and provide the body with the requirements for health is the first step towards wellness. Disease processes are not reversed with medication or other potions. The *materia medica* consists of remedies for diseases that also produce disease. A complete transformation in the mode of living, by eliminating harmful influences, creates health. Disease occurs as a result of the body deprived and poisoned, and depends also on the genetic strength and weakness. Interfering with the healing process complicates disease and prevents optimum health.

> Dr. Trall, M.D., in his lecture to the Smithsonian Institution, in Washington, D.C., 1880, stated: "I would reject drugs if there were no other remedial agents in the universe, because, if I could do no good, I would 'cease to do evil.' I would not poison a person because he is sick."

Taking into account the factors affecting the whole organism will determine the proper care of the individual. Lifestyle modification, by supplying the conditions for health and removing harmful influences, allow the organism to heal itself. This can take anywhere from days or months to years, depending on previous living. Problems that do not respond to change of lifestyle respond best to fasting. Fasting provides strength to the physical, mental and spiritual needs of the body.

The fountain of youth is within. The power to create health and a perfect equilibrium is inherent in every organism. The processes of construction and destruction, waste and repair are necessary to attain wellness. "Due to the weakness and deterioration, waste accumulates during the entire life period of the body." (Dr. Herbert Shelton, Vol. L, *Orthobionomics*, 1972, p. 291) Fasting eliminates the waste as all body functions are at rest.

Cause and effect is an infallible principle in nature. Modern science has to believe that nature is never wrong. True science researches the true art of healing, which is found in nature. A fast provides purification for the whole body. Due to lack of exercise, denatured foods, lack of fresh air, sunlight, pure water, emotional poise, rest and proper sleep, as well as relaxation and productivity, the body is unable to digest and eliminate to its full capacity. Un-eliminated waste products accumulate in the cells, tissues and organs, as a result of this poor body management; and the internal environment will be the attraction for any specific micro-organisms. The fast is the key to eternal youth and the secret to perfect and permanent health. Fasting is nature's safety valve and the automatic protection against illness. Toxic wastes accumulated in the organism accelerate the aging process, causing suffering, pain and premature death. Waste that is not removed regularly thickens the blood in conjunction with products of imperfect metabolism interfering with the natural functioning of all body duties. Accumulated poisons must be eliminated by fasting in order to restore and maintain wellness. Regeneration and repair begins as blood garbage and waste are removed.

Water Flowing

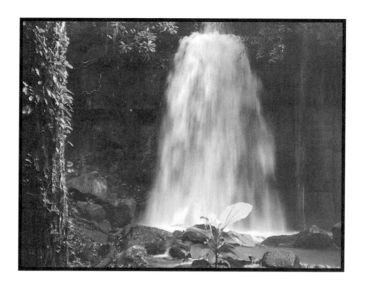

Cleansing - Healing - Purifying

CHAPTER IV

"...and you shall be like a watered garden like a spring that never runs dry..."

Garden

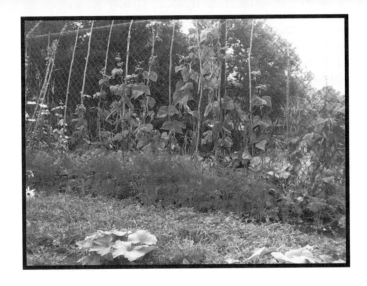

FASTING FOR HEALTH AND DISEASE

NATURE'S WAY OF PURIFICATION AND TRANSFORMATION

Fasting has been practiced since primitive man began to search for food. Today human beings forsake food to lose weight or to save money. Fasting is the key to eternal youth and the secret to perfect and permanent health. Abstaining from food and drinking pure water is the valid means of restoring and preserving health, and a useful tool for change, but not survival.

The origin of the word "fasting" comes from the old English word, "fiesting, "meaning" to be disciplined or strict." Fasting is not drinking juice, or eliminating certain kinds of foods. It is the voluntary abstinence from all food and unlike any notion of starvation. During a fast the body lives off stored reserves of food.

Religious fasts were common throughout history. This was done in atonement for sin, in self-denial, prior to making important decisions, or as a form of prayer and thanksgiving. Animals in nature fast when wounded or sick. "It is known that spiders will go 18 to 24 months without any intake of food. The transformations from tadpole to frog, caterpillar to butterfly, are "autolytic," or disintegrative, self-digesting acts, or fasting states, a remarkable feat of creating an entirely different organism." (Dr. Frank Sabatino, Lecture, Sept. 1987) "A dog or cat if sick or wounded will crawl under the wood shed or some secluded spot and rest until well, without taking food." (Dt. Sabatino's Lecture)

The elephant if wounded, and still able to travel, will "go along with the rest of the herd and can be found supporting himself beside a tree while the remainder of the herd enjoys a hearty meal." (Dr. Shelton, *Human Life: Its Philosophy and Laws*, 1979, p. 251) It is also known that cows or horses refuse food when sick. Fasting is an instinctual process and is lost only by humans, although the appetite is curbed when illness is experienced. Often it is heard that one must eat to keep up one's strength. Humans are the only animals who continue to eat when ill.

In nature, there are many instances of fasting: "Salmon swimming upstream battle currents during spawning season – in the fasting state. The queen ant leaves her colony, mates with a male, digs a hole in the ground and starts to dissolve her wings. The dissolved wing muscle will autolyze and be used as nutrients. She will have larvaes, care for them alone for months and still feed herself with a small amount of her saliva and leftover parts from the wing muscle." (Dr. Sabatino, *The Journal*, Sept. 1987, p. 8) Patients stuffed with food and the promptings of nature's instinctual messages prolong the illness and complicate the healing process. It is important to realize that when there is no hunger, there will be no digestion; therefore, food must be withheld. Undigested food putrefies, ferments and causes toxic substances to be emitted into the bloodstream.

Fasting is feared and misunderstood by many today. Those suspicious have never fasted, nor have they any knowledge or experience in the subject. Fasting is an instinctive quality in animal life, and it is also instinctive to humans who have been fasting for centuries. When a patient is ill, the desire to eat diminishes, yet they are encouraged to eat for strength.

The human digestive tract is somewhere between twenty-five and thirty feet long. The body requires time to process the complex material consumed each day into something it can use for energy and vitality. Each cell is lined with mucous and a variety of enzymes, as well as having a backup digestive system.

In water-only fasting, nutrition does not come to a halt even though food is not consumed. In metabolism, blood sugar provides nutrition to the brain and nervous system. It is important that blood sugar levels are normal and basic at all times. There are three ways the body provides this basic level of blood sugar at all times. When food is eaten, a certain amount of it keeps blood sugar levels normal. When more food is consumed than the body requires, the extra nutrients are stored for future use. The body creates glycogen, which is stored in the liver, and this is like a by-product created from starches. When more is eaten than can be stored in the liver and bloodstream, then the body still holds on to it and the body takes the sugar and converts it into proteins and fats. (Dr. Sabatino, Conference, 1985)

When one stops eating, the first thing that happens is that blood sugar drops. The body leans on the glycogen reserves in a conservative fashion. The body also takes fats and proteins and makes them into sugars. This is known as gluconeogenesis. So the body takes fats and proteins and makes them into sugars. In fasting, the body begins to burn off fat tissue. The body prefers at this time to use protein to make sugar. The body takes fatty acids, the basic building blocks of fats, and the brain shifts where it begins to burn up the source of energy.

One of the by-products of fat metabolism is called ketones. During a fast, ketosis develops and is shown in the darker urine, the foul breath and perspiration during the fast. In the past many believed that the ketones would destroy the kidneys and create acidosis and waste the body away. This is a great misconception about fasting. This shift the brain makes allows the body to be able to fast safely. This spares the protein and uses fat metabolism, which maintains the energy of the system. (Dr. Sabatino, Fasting Tape, 1994) Proteins are not broken down, as is indicated in urine tests, and very little nitrogen is excreted. Scientific research done in fasting institutions have proven the constructive value of fasting, as well as its safety for the human organism. Fears of fasting are based on this one particular concern, that of using up important amino acids.

The mind and body are in unity, and during a fast one can experience emotional as well as physiological changes. Dr. Yuri Nikolayev of the Moscow Psychiatric Institute, director of the fasting unit, has experienced a breakthrough in the treatment of schizophrenia: When all other treatment and therapy failed, fasting corrected the biochemical imbalances. "Many would have deteriorated and lived out the balance of their lives in the bleak back wards of a mental hospital. Seventy percent of those treated by fasting improved so remarkably that they were able to resume an active life." (Dr. Alan Cott, M.D., *Fasting: The Ultimate Diet*, Bantum Books, 1975, p. 34)

The body in its wisdom begins to use what it needs least during a fast, to provide what it needs most. This means that the organism is provided with stored nutritive substances to nourish the body wherever it is needed, and the body removes and dissolves unnecessary substances, as well as it dissolves tumors, cysts, and growths in order to keep its integrity. (Dr. Sabatino, Regency Spa, Sept. 1991) Waste products are moved out rapidly and fat cells throw more waste into the system. There is an increased amount of activity in all the eliminative organs, such as the liver, kidneys, heart, skin, and lungs, as well as in all cells, tissues, and organs, discharging accumulated, stored excrement. The fat cells serve as a garbage dump for waste. Fasting, being a constructive process of purification, takes care of all uneliminated waste very rapidly; and the patient will observe this in certain symptoms, such as headaches, certain dream activity, aches and pains; and what may seem like a destructive illusion is the body's vitality trying to purify itself and restore all body functions back to normal.

Due to the symptoms experienced during a fast, some may be disillusioned in thinking that during this crisis the body is not healing but getting worse, yet there is a specific reason for the crisis. It is important to emphasize here to fast under careful supervision, so that during a healing crisis fear and misinterpretation of what is happening can be explained by an expert, and the patient is supported during this time. There is much fear associated with the vitality of the body during a fast. Even though there is weakness during a fast, the primary source of energy comes from fatty tissue. There is a misconception about fasting and the use of protein tissue and self-digestion during a fast. The body keeps its integrity during the fast, providing the fast is properly supervised, studied and learned from by a doctor or a person trained in supervising fasts. "People don't realize that the chief obstacle to fasting is in overcoming the cultural and social and psychological fears of going without food. These fears are ingrained." (Alan Cott, M.D. *Fasting as a Way of Life*, 1977, p. 53, quoting, in a taped conversation, Dr. Charles Goodrich, Mount Sinai School of Medicine, N.Y., who has fasted many times).

FASTING IS NOT STARVATION

Fasting is a constructive and conservative process of allowing the body a physiological rest and leaning on reserved nutrients to nourish and supply bodily needs. When the body goes beyond the reserved tissue and one continues to fast, then the body begins to go through starvation. In the fasting state the body is supported and constructive symptoms of physiology are noted. Blood pressure drops rapidly, pulse is stable, the system is calm. Protein levels are maintained and blood chemistry is consistent, breathing is normal. Dr. George F. Cahill, Jr. of Harvard Medical School has noted: "Man's survival (of long abstentions from food) is predicated upon the remarkable ability to conserve the relatively limited body protein stores while utilizing fat as the primary energy-producing food." (Alan Cott, M.D. *Fasting as a Way of Life*, 1977, p. 57)

It is stated that in going beyond the body's reserves, certain symptoms are noticed: The pulse becomes rapid, blood pressure drops and continues to drop, and it usually takes a long fast to experience these symptoms. Fasting is a positive, orderly process, constructive and healing. Starvation is derived from the word "sterben," meaning, "to die." Fasting is voluntary and healing; starvation is involuntary and the individual is deprived of nourishment and it is destructive, noticeable in the physiology of the body.

WHY FAST

Modern society provokes the body with vitamins, minerals, drugs, coffee, devitalized foods and stimulants. The body becomes depressed to the same extent that it was stimulated and it goes through a withdrawal syndrome. At this point the individual uses more nerve energy than the body has available. The body is pushed beyond its capacity to build and repair; and during the fast the body, in its constructive effort to restore and rejuvenate itself, pays a price. The person who abuses the body and over stimulates the system becomes extremely toxic and feels the discomfort during the fast. The illusion that stimulants give energy can be more noticeable during the fast. The vitality of the body during the fast will show up strongly with headaches, pain, discomfort, and sometimes vomiting, which eventually disappear as the fast progresses.

The physiological rest that fasting provides can sometimes mean for some people being in bed and resting, while for others, it may mean cutting out light, reading, TV, radio, and all activity. The fast is the only valid means of restoring the body back to balance. With modern society's food and environmental pollution, as well as the stress individuals experience, it is necessary to fast so that stored waste material can be eliminated and the body's cells, tissues, organs, and fluids can be restored to normal.

THE FASTING METHOD—LIFE EXPERIENCES

It is logical to fast when ill because nature tells us to do this. When acute disease is experienced, the patient is tired, and the appetite disappears. To eat at this time is to die and to abstain is to live. Dr. Walter, in *Life's Great Law*, p. 209, says, "No process of treatment ever invented fulfills so many indications of restoration of health as does fasting. It is nature's own primal process, her first requirement in nearly all cases, promoting circulation, improving nutrition, facilitating excretion, recuperating vital power, and restoring vital vigor, it has no competitor." (*The Journal*, Aug. 1984) To rest the organs of digestion is of great importance and rewards the patient with comfort and a speedy recovery.

It is not that fasting is a cure for disease, but is a restorative process. Dr. Jennings, one of the greatest pioneers in the health field, says, "It is of no advantage to urge food upon the stomach when there is no digestive power to work it up. There is never any danger of starvation so long as there are reserved forces sufficient to hold the citadel of life."(Jennings, quoted by Dr. Shelton in *Human Life: Its Philosophy and Laws*, 1979, p. 252) When nutrients are required by the body, the digestive power will become efficient and a voracious appetite will return. If no food is taken in acute disease, recovery takes place rapidly and suffering ceases. The body lives off the reserves stored over many months, provided the individual practiced a healthy lifestyle. "These nutritive reserves are ready for use at short notice and with little energy expenditure by the body. They are capable of supplying all essential needs for the time being, and can be replenished at leisure, after the work of reconstruction has been completed." (Shelton, *Human Life*, p, 254)

The body continues to repair and grow tissue, etc., during a fast. Some examples of this are: Dr. Oswald records a case of a young dog that fell from a high barn loft and broke two legs and three ribs and injured his lungs. He refused all food except water for twenty days … Not until the twenty-sixth day would he take meat. The bones knit, the lungs healed and the dog was able to run and bark as before." (Shelton, *Human Life*, p. 254) Also, "the growth of granulation tissues in wounds continues during the deepest slumber." It is also noted that growths and tumors shrink during a fast: "Tumor-like growths are often rapidly absorbed and large tumors are reduced in size." (Shelton, p. 255) Diseases of various kinds are eliminated during a fast: "Diseased tissues are broken down, exudates, effusions, and deposits are absorbed and eliminated." The brain and nervous system benefit during a fast. "The brain and nervous system are supported and lose no weight during a fast, while the less important tissues are sacrificed to feed them." (Shelton, p. 255)

Insanity, nervous symptoms, and mental powers are improved during a fast. An extremely nervous lady fasted only one week and, "her nervousness was completely overcome in this short time." (Shelton p. 255)

Mental improvement is experienced during a fast, as well as intuition, sympathy, and love; and intellectual and emotional qualities are given a new life. "Fasting does increase one's control over all his appetites and passions." (Shelton, p. 256)

Quantities of blood and nervous energy are used by the digestive system to help digest a meal. During a fast the mind becomes clearer, the senses more acute, and the faster experiences a certain euphoria. As one no longer is an addict to food and drink, the body has a chance to purify and restore itself to balance. One case of hearing impairment restored during a fast:

"Catarrhal deafness of long standing, where there are no adhesions in the Eustachian tube, is always improved or overcome. People who have been deaf for years are enabled to hear the ticking of a watch and low sounds that before were impossible." (Shelton, p. 256)

An example of taste and smell being restored: "I have seen the senses of taste and smell, which had been long paralyzed, restored to their normal condition while fasting." (Shelton, p. 256)

Eyesight becomes restored to normal after a fast: "People who have worn glasses for years and who could not read without them are frequently enabled by a fast to discard their glasses and find their sight to be better than before. The eyes also become clear and bright." (Shelton, p. 256)

Dr. Shelton points out how the senses become deadened because of depleted "vitality and the accumulation in the tissues of excess food and retained waste matter."

An important fact is noted about how the blood improves during a fast. "This increase of erythrocytes, during the early part of the fast, he regarded as due to improved nutrition resulting from a cessation of overeating. This increase in red blood cells has been noted even in anemia." (Shelton, p. 256) Reported results by Senator and Mueller note that "after a short period of diminution in the number of red blood corpuscles there is a slight increase, also, that the number of white blood corpuscles decrease as the fast progresses, and, the number of eosinophils and polynuclear cells increases, as well as that the alkalinessence of blood diminishes." (Shelton, p. 257)

The liver, kidneys and spleen receive a greater supply of nervous energies because of rest, and the work of elimination from these organs is enhanced, and as well any damage or weakness heals quickly. "Since no food is consumed, they are allowed an opportunity to catch up with the work of purification." (Shelton, p. 257)

During a fast the bowels take a rest. "Sometimes they will continue to move for the first three or four days of the fast and in some instances diarrhea will develop … starving shipwrecked men had not had a movement for twenty and thirty days." Dr. Shelton disapproved of using enemas and did not employ this practice at his San Antonio Health School. He believed that during the rest, the stomach and colon repaired and restored themselves to normal.

Dr. Shelton quotes Mr. Carrington, who discovered lungs heal more than any other organ: "Lung tissue possesses the inherent power of healing itself in a far shorter time … than any other organ which may be diseased." (Shelton, p. 258)

All secretions in the body become normal and the foul smell associated with them is diminished. The more toxic the body, the more foul the smell.

There is a gain in strength during a fast. The first few days are difficult and the faster may be lethargic and low in energy. "As paradoxical as it may seem to those who have had no experience with fasting, there is a frequent, and perhaps always, a gain in strength while fasting." After the body has a chance to eliminate the stored waste material, vitality is noticed as the fast progressed. "Others record numerous examples of increase of both mental and physical strength during the fast." (Shelton, p. 259) The purity of the blood is what measures strength in muscles and nerves.

"Fasting brings about the purification of the blood and also conserves nervous energy, so that there is more energy on hand to be used and the condition of nerve and muscle is improved so that they respond more readily to the will … the increase in strength is most marked in those who are most toxic and overloaded with excess food." (Shelton, p. 259)

It is important to note that the heart is strengthened during a fast to a great degree. Dr. Shelton quotes Mr. Carrington from his book, *Vitality, Fasting and Nutrition*, p. 464:

"The fact that weak hearts are actually strengthened and cured by fasting proves conclusively that unusual symptoms observed during this period denote a beneficial reparative process, and not any harmful or dangerous decrease, due to a lack of perfect control by the cardiac nerve." (Shelton, p. 259)

The feeling of weakness during the fast is something most individuals find very difficult. It is due to the withdrawal of the accustomed stimulants, as well as the body working excessively to remove deeply stored toxins. "As the fast progresses he will feel stronger and more cheerful. Fainting during the fast usually comes, if at all, during these first three or four days." (Shelton, p. 259)

The pulse rate varies during a fast and could go up to 120 or drop as low as 40. Changes in the pulse denote changes taking place in the body, such as "weak hearts are actually strengthened and cured by fasting … proves a beneficial reparative process…" Extremes in the pulse rate do not denote any danger from the fast and are symptoms of a healing crisis. (Shelton, p. 260)

The temperature during a fast could rise or fall, although most persons experience a normal body temperature. A sense of chilliness is felt throughout the fast because of a "decreased cutaneous circulation … If we cannot fast without fever, it is because we have been previously improperly fed." (Shelton, p. 260)

One of the most important successes of fasting has been in the area of hypertension. While fasting, blood pressure drops quickly because the heart rate slows and the body is calm and resting. When the heart slows, blood pressure drops rapidly. In chronic hypertension, "hypertension is reduced in a few days … even one day in a fast." ("Fasting," *The Journal*, Sept. 1987, p. 10) Also, fasting has a positive effect on insulin resistance; meaning that when insulin is adequate, but it is "ineffective due to resistance at the cells, in the liver and elsewhere, your blood sugar levels rise. This can lead to serious clinical consequences. Fortunately, after a period of fasting, this problem is often dramatically improved."

Dr. Frank Sabatino also states that individuals lose three to five times more sodium from the tissues than in any other state. Sodium makes people retain fluid and with fluid loss, blood volume drops; also blood pressure drops and thyroid slows. Blood, thyroid and metabolic changes all are unique parts of the fasting state. ("Fasting," *The Journal*, Sept. 1987, p. 10)

The body produces excess, harmful poisons when sodium and fluids are retained, by the decomposition of carbohydrates, fats, and proteins, which are absorbed into the blood stream, causing toxemia. Health cannot be synchronized out of poison; and the sick need helpful things, not hurtful things, to get well. Fasting helps to cleanse and purify the entire system and removes the cause of illness. These poisons must be removed through fasting, so they are not allowed to accumulate in the cells, tissues, and organs. Waste must be excreted as quickly as it is accumulated because it is deadly and interferes with healthy functioning.

Fasting cleanses the arteries and improves blood circulation, high blood pressure, and can reverse heart disease. In an article published in the June 2001 issue of *The Journal of Manipulative and Physiological Therapeutics*, entitled "Medically Supervised Water Fasting in the Treatment of Hypertension," Dr. Colin Campbell, world-renowned nutritionist and biochemist of Cornell University, who has done much in this field of healthy lifestyle, presented the article introduced to him by Dr. Alan Goldhamer, of True North Health Center, to his senior research associate, who was impressed with the findings and co-authored the study. In an article in *Health Science*, Fall, 2001, Mark Epstein has stated that as a result of the article and successes in fasting, the International Union of Operating Engineers has made fasting a fully covered medical benefit to any current or retired member or spouse, and it is noted that over half of the members have diabetes or hypertension. Also, as a result of the recent successes through fasting, the State of Nevada has recently approved fasting as a medical benefit. These organizations have realized that because of the rise in cost of medical care, fasting can provide health benefits. Fasting has proved to be important in improving health care costs.

It is also known that when blood volume drops during fasting, the vessels become smaller, more resistant, and sodium is lost due to the retention of fluids and salts; this drops the blood pressure.

The thyroid slows down because the metabolic rate slows down and the glands secrete less. Water balance is corrected very rapidly. The hormonal system slows down and metabolic changes occur because digestion is halted, and the body can deal with healing all these changes. There are also neurological changes. In this state of rest, the energy of the body is used and is available wherever it is most needed, to the whole organism. Fasting is profound elimination and shows up in the body's vitality in trying to detoxify and clean the areas of uric acid, cholesterol, PCBs, and many other toxic chemical residues.

Most important, to initiate the drastic cleansing process that fasting provides, it is of utmost importance to rest and remain free of work, stress, worry, gossip, and anxiety.

WHAT TO EXPECT DURING A FAST—AND HOW TO KNOW IT IS COMPLETE

After the third day of fasting the appetite and desire for food disappears, unless an individual has had a large supply of stimulants prior to the fast. The return of hunger is an indication that the fast has come to an end and food is to be introduced slowly. Starvation begins at this point, if no food is consumed. When the body is hungry and requires food, and nourishment is not supplied, starvation begins. At this point all reserves have been utilized by the body during the fast and the body is ready to eat with true hunger. "Mr. Carrington and others insist on carrying the fast to completion, that is, until the return of natural hunger." (Shelton, *Human Life: Its Philosophy and Laws*, 1979, p. 261) These are some valuable indications to help us to know when the fast is completed:

- The tongue becomes clean
- The breath becomes sweet
- The body temperature becomes normal
- The salivary secretion is resumed
- The bad taste in the mouth ends
- The eyesight becomes clear and sharp and the eyes bright
- The excreta becomes odorless
- There is a return of hunger felt in the throat and mouth just as thirst becomes genuine (Shelton, *Human Life*, p. 271)

It is important to understand that healing crises will be experienced during the fast, and that one allows the crisis to happen. No longer will the crisis be masked with potions and drugs, and this vitality creates healing.

WHY NOT TO FAST

There are many causes of impaired elimination. Overeating is one of them; others are improper food, such as processed and junk foods, cooked foods, salt, sugar, and other poisons such as pesticides and fungicides, alcohol, drugs, chocolate, caffeine, tea, and other stimulants and chemicals, such as spices, soda pop, and other substances that enervate and impair excretion. One can say that everyone today needs to fast to correct and change the body and bring it back to normal. There are certain conditions that do not respond well to fasting: certain kinds of cancer that have metastasized to a particular organ, such as the liver, or pancreatic cancer and certain types of heart disease. Very thin people need to have time to build up reserves before fasting, or should fast for only a few days to aid metabolism.

It is wise to be checked by a knowledgeable doctor before fasting and not to fast on one's own but to seek professional help. If an individual is unable to fast, then an improved dietary plan can correct a clogged system somewhat. It may take longer, but the body does respond well to an improved nutritional plan. Well-regulated and systematic exercises are important in prevention and maintaining health.

WHEN TO FAST

When the desire for food is diminished and the body is experiencing a healing crisis, or any acute disease, such as a fever, cold, or flu, this is the time to listen to the body and take control. Hippocrates, the first physician, said, "To eat when you are sick is to feed the sickness."

It is best to fast in the summer when it is warm, as the body feels chilled very easily during a fast. Dr. Shelton suggests, "Not to delay the fast because of the temperature outside because the temperature of a faster usually rises, but to fast when it is necessary." (Shelton, *Science and Fine Art of Fasting*, 1978, p. 252)

Dr. Shelton also suggests that if there are negative symptoms during pregnancy, such as nausea, vomiting, lack of appetite and other symptoms, the woman ought to fast; also if it is necessary during lactation, but only under careful supervision, as it stops the secretion of milk. (Shelton, *Science and Fine Art of Fasting*, p. 256) The milk supply will return quickly after the fast.

The elderly do well with a fast, but they need to be supervised and the fast is usually a short one. Those who are fearful about fasting ought not to fast until they fully understand it and are comfortable with a fast. A fast is a peaceful, calm experience and one must be convinced that it is good and be relaxed about it.

When an individual decides to fast it is important that the diet is cleaned up so that the fast is a pleasant experience. Raw fruits and vegetables are beneficial prior to the fast. They provide fiber so that elimination is improved. These foods are high in water content and are potent factors in "liquefying excretions in the tissues," thus promoting drainage of protein and carbohydrate waste. Raw nuts and seeds and whole grains and steamed vegetables can also be adapted in moderation before the fast. (Shelton, *Health Review*)

Avoiding stimulants of all kinds, such as alcohol, tobacco, caffeine, chocolate, sugars, pop, etc., prior to a fast helps to create better balance, sounder sleep and less anxiety during a fast.

HOW LONG TO FAST

Some individuals who experience extreme weakness may have to do short fasts only. This also applies to those who are emaciated. If there is extreme degeneration, a series of short fasts, under supervision, with correct nutritional guidance, may be beneficial. "In the latter stages of consumption and cancer, the fast can be of no value except to relieve the patient's suffering ... fasting is of distinct benefit in the earlier stages of both of these conditions." (Shelton, *Fasting Can Save Your Life*, p. 248)

It is important to have supervision during a fast because the doctor knows how long the fast ought to be and when it is right to complete. To ensure that the fast can continue without any complications, and can continue safely, it is of great concern not to break a fast during a healing crisis; that the blood pressure is monitored daily; and that the tongue, pulse, heart, urine, and blood are monitored.

HOW TO BREAK A FAST

How to break a fast will depend on how long one fasts. It is customary to have at least two days of just drinking fresh fruit and vegetable juices—that is 8 ounces of freshly made live juice every two hours from approximately 8:30 am to 5:30 pm.

Juices recommended also depend on the person's condition before and during the fast. Introducing watermelon juice, using some of the rind, is a good one to begin. After that, any of these combinations in equal portions are good:

- golden delicious apple, celery, and carrot
- carrot, lettuce, and celery
- carrot, beet, and cucumber
- carrot, spinach, and celery

Juices are to be sipped very slowly and water is to be taken as thirst demands. It is most important that the fast be broken when the person is stable and not experiencing a healing crisis.

After two days of juice the foods given for breakfast, lunch, and supper are to be fresh, whole, live and raw. For instance, fresh fruit for breakfast; fresh fruits, lettuce, celery and cucumber for lunch; and a combination salad for supper.

Slowly introduce nuts, seeds, and nut butters for lunch and an avocado for supper.

The appetite after a few days becomes voracious and one must take care not to overeat but to eat lightly and to introduce other foods slowly. Eating in moderation is of great importance.

There are many ways of cleansing and rejuvenating the body, yet fasting on water only is the most therapeutic and effective.

Other cleanses that help those who cannot fast on water only are juices as above mentioned, or just eating fresh fruits and vegetables for breakfast, lunch, and supper, and adding juices before meals, thus avoiding all concentrated starches and proteins. This will not be as beneficial, yet it may help those who are feeble and not capable of a water fast. For those with weak digestion and who suffer from the loss of their teeth, blended salads and raw blended soups are recommended.

DOCTORS SPECIALIZING IN FASTING

Alec Burton, M.Sc. D.O. D.C. and
Neijla Burton, D.O.
Arcadia Health Centre,
Cobah Road, Arcadia, N.S.W.
2159 Australia
Phone: 011-61-2653-1115

Frank Sabatino, D.C. PhD
Regency House Natural Health Spa
2000 S. Ocean Drive
Hallandale, FL 33009
Phone: (954) 454-2220

D.J. Scott, D.C.
Scott's Natural Health Institute
17023 Lorain Ave.
Cleveland, OH 44111 60
Phone: (216) 671-5023

Joel Fuhrman, M.D.
450 Amwell Rd.
Belle Mead, NJ 08502
Phone: (908) 359-1775

Alan Goldhamer, DC
True North Health
1551 Pacific Avenue
Santa Rosa, Ca
95404
Phone: (707) 586-5555
www.healthpromoting.com

Natures Health
Halanna Matthew, PhD
Vancouver, BC Canada
(604) 926-3009
info@natureshealthltd.com

TESTIMONIALS FROM FASTERS

Hippocrates, the first medicine man, said. "Fasting combats disease." Dr. Yuri Nikolayev, having fasted over 10,000 people with very serious diseases, says, "Fasting allows the body to mobilize its defense mechanisms against many illnesses, and healing being a biological process, allows the digestive system to rest, creating healing of body, mind and soul." (Alan Cott, M.D., *Fasting as a Way of Life*, p. 4) Remarkable healing takes place during a fast as the individual surrenders to the messages of the body and adheres to the discipline of fasting.

Dr. Herbert M. Shelton (1895-1985), teacher, writer, researcher, doctor in many fields, almost single-handedly delved and probed into the storehouse of knowledge of the early pioneer doctors in many fields of health and brought to the world the philosophy and science behind fasting. Having fasted himself and thousands of people at his San Antonio Health School, he had the experience, research, and wisdom to write books and articles on fasting, from which we have learned.

A young athlete fasted at Dr. Shelton's Health School for forty-six days after a severe injury that doctors said required surgery. He refused this and fasted instead. At the end of the fast he was able to walk again.

Joe, who was requested by his doctor to undergo five by-passes, did not want to go this route. In this situation, he could only cleanse his body with fresh live vegetable juices, since he was on medication for over five years. After following a dietary change, drinking fresh juices, beginning to slowly exercise, and having short fasts, he went to his doctor, who was amazed and requested that he continue to do what he was doing because after approximately seven months his arteries were clear and open. This patient was also 80% deaf in one ear and now enjoys 100% hearing.

Maria wanted to have a son but her doctor advised her she needed to have a hysterectomy because of excessive bleeding. A relative who was a medical doctor advised her to get another opinion, as he did not think she should have this drastic operation. Maria wrote this letter after she made some healthy dietary changes and undertook a short juice and water fast: "After a fast of three or four days and changing my dietary habits to more healthier ones, I did not have to have a hysterectomy and now have a son."

Joan had digestive problems and decided to fast under proper supervision for seven days. She went through some healing crises during the week and stayed in bed much of the time, except for the occasional walk. At the end of the fast she began to be free of discomfort and was able to take juice. A short while after the fast she said she was sleeping much better and digesting well.

Vicky had a bad case of arthritis and her fingers began to swell, twist, and ache. After one week of water-only fasting, the pain was gone; the swelling and extreme arthritic condition healed. Her fingers became close to normal. Seven months later she is still experiencing the benefits of her fast. Her lifestyle has changed to a plant-based diet with little fruit and many vegetables.

Another woman, who had been given much medication for panic attacks, then depression, then high blood pressure, overcame treating all the symptoms when she was able to fast and then eat a balanced nutritional diet. She says this: "Did I ever thank you from the bottom of my heart for rescuing me from my lower self that had taken over my life? There are really no words that can describe my deepest gratitude and my love for you. The way you cared for me for two weeks in full, will never be forgotten. I am now almost six months sober and have not taken any medication!!! A wondrous journey indeed, that has brought me back to a close relationship with my 'kind Father' — my beloved God and His Angels. Love and thanks forever..." *Christina*

Reece worked for the construction company that renovated one of the homes I lived in. I noticed he was leaning against the house often throughout the day so I invited him to share how he was feeling. He said that he was diagnosed with colitis and was given blood infusions every month because of low blood. He asked if he could eat lunch with us so he could get used to better ways of eating. He began to feel better. He asked for a dietary plan to take home and in a short time felt he no longer needed the gamma infusions. To this day, Reece calls to say that he is feeling more energy and vitality, and he went back to school to graduate from a Fine Arts Program. He did not fast but followed a healthier lifestyle with optimum results.

Dr. Frank McCoy's book, *The Fast Way to Health* (McCoy Publications Inc., 1926, Los Angeles), contains several cases of individuals healed through fasting.

McCoy says, "Disease is not accidental but is caused in every case by destructive habits. Bad habits of thought, insufficient exercise, and innumerable other errors of life must be considered as contributing causes, but above all, dietetic mistakes must be corrected." Dr. McCoy stresses the importance of fasting to eliminate the "morbid material in organs or tissues of the body." In his many years of practice, he states, "I have made the most exhaustive study of every method of cure to modern surgery and gland therapy, and I have never found a single method that could approach even closely, in its results, the benefits which come from some form of the fasting cure." He also gives a definition of fasting as "restriction of food and drink" and states, "Fasting gives the body a chance to cleanse itself of the accumulation of the products of imperfect metabolism due to the over-ingestion of food which the body could not use for building or repair material." (p. 17)

Listed below are some of the success stories Dr. McCoy experienced:

> "A boy six years of age with asthma, wheezing since a few days after birth, which kept him awake at night, fasted for three days on a fast of small amounts of orange juice and water. With a well-balanced diet after the fast the child slept eleven or twelve hours every night and has not had a re-occurrence of asthma. (p. 39)

> "A young woman thirty-five years of age suffering from severe pains in the lower back, who had taken treatments with no relief, fasted for twelve days using large quantities of water. Her backache was being caused by a bladder, which was being constantly irritated by urine overloaded with poisonous material that the liver had been unable to

eliminate in the form of bile. After this was completed, a well-balanced diet was resumed and she was advised to avoid foods tending to cause biliousness, which enlarged her gall bladder, causing inflammation of the bladder and in turn causing her backache.

"A man, thirty-five years of age with serious psoriasis since a small boy, fasted for thirty-two days and at the end of that time the skin was almost entirely clear. All the hair on his body had been removed by the disease and was restored.

"A woman twenty-eight years of age with a large fibroid tumor partially protruding from the vagina and about the size of a large grapefruit, having the stomach and intestines prolapsed and lying upon the fibroid, being pushed downward by the weight, started a fast of twenty-eight days. By this time three-fourths of the tumor had been removed by the power of the fast."

Dr. McCoy explains how the overeating of all kinds of foods, the use of improper combinations of foods, too many carbohydrates, and the use of gassy foods, such as onions, garlic, cooked cabbage, dry beans, etc., cause inflammation, growths, poor circulation and a multitude of problems, such as insomnia, aches and pains, prolapses, sagging organs, and sickness. (McCoy, *Fast Way to Health*, 1926, p.1-323)

Dr. Joel Fuhrman, M.D., points out how effective fasting is in the recovery of diabetes, a disease that is destroying many lives, causing premature death, disability and suffering. In adult-onset diabetes, he says, "More recent studies reporting on fasting of diabetic patients have … shown excellent results and confirm the changes … following a prolonged fast, the diabetic patient shows a substantial improvement in insulin function independent of the degree of weight loss, and restoration of pancreatic function can occur that does not occur with weight loss alone. Complete remission of diabetes was reported in many patients ... Fasting should not be used early in the treatment, but rather after many months of the diabetic reversal diet, when the person has lost most of the excessive weight." (Dr. Furhman, *Fasting and Eating for Health*, First St. Martin's Edition, May 1998, p. 139)

Autoimmune disease is a major problem today, leaving people crippled and taking a multitude of harmful medications; many derive positive relief from fasting. Dr. Furhman says, "The majority of cases respond to fasting and plant-based diets. It is predictable that in spite of well-conducted scientific investigations and the clinical experience of many physicians the effective nutritional treatment for autoimmune disease is ignored ... optimum nutrition alone can prevent the suffering of millions. Fasting is a remarkable anti-inflammatory intervention, more powerful than the strongest and most toxic drugs at reducing inflammation." (Furhman, p. 144 and 154) The fast suppresses the pain and stops the deterioration of the joints and body, as well as improves digestion, which is a problem for most arthritic sufferers.

Dr. Fuhrman has had results with lupus through fasting. "After a twenty-day fast in 1992, the patient was placed on a low-fat, low protein diet devoid of dairy products ... all the lupus symptoms had resolved." (p. 160)

Ulcerative colitis and Crohn's disease are inflammatory diseases involving the lining of the intestines. The disease responds well to a modification in dietary habits, as well as to fasting. One of Dr. Fuhrman's patients who fasted had a family history of colitis. "She fasted for three weeks to place the disease in remission. Now she undergoes an extended fast every few years to ensure that she maintains her remission." (p. 168)

FASTING AS CONTROVERSIAL

Recently the California Medical Board has filed a formal complaint with the California Chiropractic Board, which is now investigating the recommendation of fasting by chiropractors. This is a challenge to health care freedom because this could mean that every doctor in the United States would be prohibited from using water fasting.

Individuals have fasted at home alone without sufficient knowledge of the science and fine art of fasting, and have ended up in hospital, or under medical care with great suspicion as to its validity. Doctors speak of fasting as "dangerous," yet harmful drugs are used. Fasting is looked upon as destructive because of symptoms experienced with the vitality of the body in expelling waste, yet it is the most constructive process, whereby reserves stored in the body are used to nourish the body during the fast. It is more destructive to allow the body to retain stored excrement for any length of time, as this leads to serious disease.

A fast must be supervised by a qualified individual who can monitor blood pressure, urine, pulse, and whatever else is necessary during a fast.

There are many fears associated with fasting because of lack of education and a lack of experience in doing it. Ignorance and misunderstanding keeps fasting controversial.

In *Environmental Nutrition*, May 1997, Vol. 20, Issue 5, p. 7, the answers on the safety and effectiveness of fasting as a way to cleanse the body of toxic waste, and the answer in the article "Fasting for Health" offer few benefits. "We do know there is no evidence it can do either of the things, cleanse the body of toxins, or lose a few pounds. It hasn't been proven to cure anything." Dr. Jeejeebhoy, in a publication entitled *Health News*, says this on the subject of fasting: "The detoxification myth may have originated with a condition called insulin resistance. It is true that these people would feel better after a 24-hour water fast, since their blood sugar and blood pressure levels would drop slightly." He also says, "There's absolutely no evidence whatsoever that if you're starving, somehow toxins pour out of your body." Dr. Kursheed Jeejeebhoy is a professor of medicine at the University of Toronto and director of nutritional support services at St. Michael's Hospital, Toronto, Ontario, Canada. He also says, "There is no therapeutic benefit to fasting." (West Vancouver Library, West Vancouver, B.C. Canada, 2001/01/01)

These are controversial statements after the evidence over many years has indicated the powerful tool fasting is in allowing the body to heal and transform.

Although many have not been educated in knowing the true meaning of fasting, and misunderstand the nature and value of fasting as being a biological process, those who have found the healing privileges it provides know that fasting is an effective means for realizing the full potential within. The rediscovery of fasting is a great awakening for the human experience in wellness and wholeness, and will continue to be sought and practiced to the end of time.

FASTING AS REJUVENATION AND TRANSFORMATION: ALLOWING THE BODY TO HEAL ITSELF

Not to fast is to forfeit the opportunity of knowing yourself, healing body, mind, spirit and emotions, letting go of the past and stepping into a new life, a new love and transformation on every level of existence.

Fasting has been practiced since the inception of life, and it is useful to both animal and human life, in all its forms. Fasting is instinctive and used for the restoration and maintenance of life and health. Dr. Scott, who has operated a fasting clinic in Ohio for many years, has success stories of thousands of patients who found their way back to health through fasting and change. "Fasting goes back to antiquity. It has a history which is most interesting and you should study it in order to improve your confidence in it. Scientists have been studying fasting for a long, long time … and they have defined the great benefits that fasting offers." (Dr. D.J. Scott, "Unfounded Fears of Fasting," *Health Science*, Nov. 1980, p. 27)

The early practitioners used fasting, and Hippocrates recognized it "as a powerful therapeutic agent, as it conforms to the laws of nature … to eat when you are sick is to feed the sickness." Dr. Scott also says, "The most consistent finding and benefit that arises out of fasting is that there is a rejuvenescence — a restoration of youthfulness."(p. 29) "Scientists who have studied fasting have found that a forty-year-old man can fast for three weeks and be restored to the physiological level of a seventeen-year-old." (p. 29) This is a remarkable anti-aging technique since the human condition constantly searches for ways to restore youthfulness. Obedience to nature's laws prevents aging, senility, and suffering.

True knowledge about fasting is available through books written by many doctors, some of which are available at libraries nationally. Dr. Scott speaks of the faulty practices and beliefs that have destroyed health. As children, many are fed when in pain and discomfort, and later in life learn to eat and stuff themselves when unhappy, or out of sorts. "The living organism is so well designed that it is capable of living throughout a whole lifetime without one moment of disease and suffering. This is consistent with its nature, its instinct and its design." (p. 28) Individuals are conditioned to solve life's problems with food, alcohol, drugs or stimulants, overeating and sexual encounters. Over the years this becomes a way of life and indulgences become inconsistent with well-being, which intoxicate the human organism. Indulgences of this kind represent the direction of interest for people.

When this focus of feeding or drinking for relief of distress become habitual, the individual will have anxiety and fear about not eating and drinking only water.

> "Enslaved by beliefs, attitudes, feelings and actions about disease, suffering and fasting, causes much confusion and suspicion about fasting for health. When withdrawal symptoms occur, weakness, nervousness and sexless feelings, which could follow after skipping a meal, these individuals are convinced diseases are accidental and drugs and food are necessary to feel good." (p. 27)

Human beings have brought the practice of fasting out of pre-history into history and there has never been a time when the fast has been abandoned. Dr. Shelton states,

> "It would be as possible to completely abandon the fast as it would be to abandon breathing. But the fast is of value only in its physiological relations to other elements of health, such as rest, sleep, exercise, water, temperature, food, cleanliness, emotional poise." (Shelton, *Science and Fine Art of Fasting*)

To fast is to change. It is a vital process by which the living organism adjusts its means to its ends. Dr. Shelton has experienced many leaving behind their crutches, wheelchairs and canes. If one wants to find a remedy for disease, fasting is Nature's only remedy. Dr. Shelton relates what he enjoyed seeing in the change of his patients after a fast:

> "Our whole life is permeated by a spirit of love and goodwill, we develop a gentleness and kindness that are new to us. A fresh zeal enters into our relations with those around us and strength is given us to perform whatever, with cheerfulness and delight. Troubles, anxieties and cares are dissipated, for we know that our welfare is secure and on a firm basis."

Dr. John Tilden, M.D., who wrote the book *Toxemia Explained, The Basic Cause of all Disease*, claims that nothing promotes the elimination of toxins more effectively than a fast. That is, abstinence of food and drink, except for water. Using eliminative or curative type diets and beverages are not as profound as the results achieved in a short space of time as the fast does. Foods do not cure; they provide nutrients to the body. To remove the cause of disease and nourish the body the way nature intended is the fast way to health. Disease is a consequence of the violation of life's laws. The recovery of health is the consequence of a return to obedience to the natural laws – then health care can cease the search for cures and instead seek the true knowledge of the laws that govern the human being. Dr. William Esser, of Esser's Health Ranch, a fasting clinic, quotes the words of Dr. Tilden, in a lecture, March 1996. "Nature – our subconscious – has a full monopoly on the power to cure. Healing is nature's prerogative, and she cannot, if she would delegate it to doctors or the academies of medical science."

Dr. Esser also quotes Herbert Ratner, M.D., who says, "Nature is a stern teacher and disciplinarian … They are my (Mother Nature's) ways. They are good. They are wise. Follow them. I have planted the seeds of fulfillment within you. Nurture those seeds and be faithful to their growth if you would harvest bounty. A plant that has withered cannot be reclaimed."

It is a worthwhile venture to investigate and experience the extraordinary and incredible facts about the water fast.

"Then your light will blaze out like the dawn and your wound be quickly healed over."
– Isaiah 58:8

Butterfly

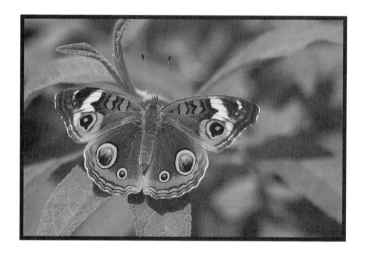

Transformation

CHAPTER V

True healing is found within.
Do no harm.
– Hippocrates

THE TRUE HEALTH CARE SYSTEM

There are two medical systems in existence: The Drug Medical System which employs poisons or chemicals, (material medica) as the proper and natural remedies for disease; the other, the Hygienic Medical System which employs normal or hygienic materials and agencies. There are several branches of the Drug Medical System, such as Allopathic, Homeopathic, Eclectic, Physio-Medical, etc., and these are essentially one and the same. They differ in certain problems and theories, but all agree in the fundamental proposition of "curing one disease by producing another." In other words, using remedies for diseases.

On the contrary, the Hygienic Medication consists in employing, as remedial agents for sick persons, the same materials and influences that preserve health in well persons. It rejects all poisons, potions, roots, barks, etc. that are incompatible with vital functions. The Hygienic System is the True System, advocating doing good by removing the cause of illness and supplying the conditions for health.

The true health care system is needed to heal the sick, suffering, and those dying prematurely. Billions of dollars are spent on campaigns, drives, and marathons to aid disease research and find cures, to no avail or support to the suffering. Education is the key. Knowledge has power and individuals are in need of correct information about health and disease.

The word "medicine" is a Latin word meaning "healing." After centuries of advertised progress, today there are more types of disease, with new names and more disability, as well as more people confused about health, than ever before. Degenerative disease is rampant, and children suffer needlessly. There is no time left to search for cures — the true health care professional must begin to help heal the suffering and teach a healthy lifestyle.

The origin of disease is no longer a mystery but a concrete fact, for which a system of education will meet and must be formulated immediately. The truth must be taught to all those interested in ministering to the sick. Through the ages, ever since the time of the ancient medical sage Hippocrates, there is evidence that only Nature ever cured anything. Nature is infallibly right all the time.

Hippocrates' oath for physicians goes back to 400 BC and says, "to abstain from whatever is harmful … and from every voluntary act of … corruption." Hippocrates lived between 400-377 BC and his motto to his colleagues was "Do No Harm." Dr. Charles E. Page, M.D., in an article on health, said that to fast means to abandon drugs and rely on nature is to correct itself. For instance, a fever is the rise of temperature designed by the body to resist and expel toxic substances, or to repair damage and is an expression of the body's enormous and inherent power to heal. This is what patients need to know — the cause of the crises. This requires going back to ancient healing methods. Five thousand years before the beginning of the Christian era, the ancient Aryan philosophers knew nothing about the synthetic preparation of drugs, and the ideal treatment involved ceasing from interfering with the body's power to heal, which brought on spontaneous recovery.

Human beings have the same nutritional needs as those of primates, that is, physiologically, anatomically, and biologically, says Dr. William Esser, who operated a Health Ranch and supervised fasts for over sixty-five years. He died August 2003, in his sleep, having never experienced sickness, and was working until almost the end. Dr. Esser confirms that primates eat all their food in the raw. Dr. Esser also states that the conditions of health never change, and it is the violation and rebellion against the laws of life that is the cause of illness.

Dr. Gerald Benesh also operated a fasting institution for approximately fifty-five years, taught nutrition and fasting, and practiced the healing arts since 1935, until close to the end of his life, which came at the age of ninety on November 15, 2002. Dr. Benesh says,

> "All cells oscillate in their own rhythm and in harmony with other cells ... each cell contains a unit of consciousness that is one with the Universal Consciousness ... uniting with all that exists. When one ponders this and comprehends the enormity of this concept, then one's consciousness changes and expands to a point where one takes on a new and more realistic perception of life. Realizing this ... creates a greater concern and respect for the living body and all that the body offers, giving one a greater incentive to live a more abundant and fulfilling life ... To do this one must comply with the Laws of Life. To deny or ignore them results in ill health, both mental and physical, ultimately ending in untimely death. The choice is ours. Learn to create the conditions for health – love and respect all life." (From a speech, "Knowing the Knower Within," Nov./Dec. 1988, Vol. III, No. 6 *The*

Journal) This explains how unified the human anatomy is and how nature complies when one cooperates with it.

Dr. Benesh was one of my most important mentors and teacher.He was able to diagnose my first child, and it was only when we began to follow his regime of having fresh live fruit and green vegetable juices, with a very simplified dietary program of fresh fruits, vegetables, nuts and seeds that the child experienced perfect health. No grains were given to young children.

My mother also came to visit us when we lived in California and had a mild case of arthritis and a cold. Dr. Benesh recommended a short supervised fast and a simplified dietary change. Her health was restored instantaneously.

When she returned home she was surprised that she could experience the sound sleep of a baby.

Dr. Benesh was reaching close to ninety and was hoping to retire. He offered for me to continue his practice. I made plans to move back to California after settling in Vancouver but due to family responsibilities was unable to take over his practice. I continued to speak to and learn from Dr. Benesh and to seek his counsel when necessary, up and until the end of his life. He had a brilliant mind, sound judgment and profound wisdom. He suffered from a car accident at the end of his life.

Dr. Scott of Scott's Natural Health Institute says we are responsible for our health. "According to the nature and design of physiology and biology of the human organism it is possible for the human to live healthfully throughout a whole lifetime … we find in this health care system that disease is not accidental – it is caused by factors most of which are environmental – most of which are avoidable and most of which are inflicted upon ourselves individually by choice and by selection – by our own activities."

A PLAN OF RESTORATION AND REJUVENATION

"There are ways of dealing with the problem of degeneration
... we must change our whole way of life."
– Dr. D.J. Scott (*Health Science*, Vol. 3 No. 3, Sept. 1980)

The new Health Care System will be a challenge to all health professionals. It will take into account the great inherent powers of the body to heal itself. It will embrace nature's laws. The laws are simple to understand. We need to teach patients the fundamental requirements of the body and how harmful influences affect the restoration of health.

We have a serious health care problem because patients are not taught how to take care of their bodies. The research must be done for the good of the patient as to the true meaning of health and disease. Wasted money, time, and effort are not providing the patient with the proper care. It is stated by eminent medical authorities that 95% of all acute illness will recover spontaneously if there is no interference to prevent the natural recovery process. No longer is the health care system to patch the human machine, but to educate more and medicate less.

The true cause of illness will be manifest in the care of the patient by supplying all the basic needs for health and eliminating all harmful influences. "All healing power is inherent in the living organism." (Shelton, Lecture, 1945) Those who are ill will experience the building up of the organism instead of a constant tearing down. This new plan teaches the patient how to remain well until his constitutional vigor declines in old age and dies from natural causes, not disease. The search for cure will now be replaced with a search to "CARE" and find out the true cause of the problem.

THE PROBLEM OF HEALTH ILLUSION

For many years people have been led to believe that health is something that just happens—something for which we are thankful but often something and we accept, but not something of which we take responsibility or take credit. Though good health is inherited to some degree, one creates health by living within the immutable laws of chemistry and physiology. The best heredity may rapidly be dissipated through unwise management of the body's powers and by exceeding the body's capabilities, or neglecting to replenish fully the body's losses. Perfect health means 100% function of every organ, tissue and cell.

The nationwide health care systems are misleading and misinforming the public about how to stop disease and become well.

Drugs mask the symptoms, suppress the disease, and are harmful, creating complications that lead to more suffering. These toxic substances are not easily eliminated and become stored in the body. Surgery, drugs, and potions do not remove the cause of disease. These treatments, the research for cures, and the technology for sustaining the ill, are all very expensive. The billions of dollars used towards finding a cure for cancer, heart disease, diabetes, arthritis, obesity, and other illnesses could be used to educate the public about how to purify and rejuvenate the body. The most treasured secret to good health and longevity, as well as to have quality living, is to keep the body clean, inside and out.

Students in medical school, nursing schools, those who care for the sick and elderly in facilities, as well as health practitioners must teach the basic principles of health so that everyone can understand how the body heals itself. Removing the cause of illness is of vital importance, as well as supplying all the conditions for health. The conditions for health are simple facts:

1. Supply the body with human nutrition based on immutable biological needs. The human organism responds best to a plant-based diet of organically grown fresh fruits and vegetables, nuts and seeds and whole grains That is all the body requires. Foods must be grown on organic soil to be adequate with the raw materials essential for human dietary needs. The foods must be picked ripe and eaten raw, in their natural state, and thoroughly masticated. These foods will provide all of the bodily nutritional needs, whether an athlete, pregnant woman, or a secretary.

2. The body is made to move and as one moves, toxins are released, the bones become strong and circulation improved. This is important for the maintenance of strength and virility.

3. Emotional poise is necessary so that worry, anxiety, fear, and negative thinking do not become part of a daily routine. Positive attitudes are constructive and lead to a feeling of happiness. When one is healthy, this comes as a normal consequence, as well as a calm and versatile countenance.

4. Rest and relaxation are necessary in order to rejuvenate and replenish nerve energy. Taking time to lay on the floor with knees up and relaxing in this comfortable position, one finds it is easy to doze for a few minutes and restore the body. Meditation is another form of rest that is powerful for the spiritual aspects of health, and equal to a good night's sleep.

5. Sleep is the great rejuvenator and it is important to have eight hours of solid sleep for adults, more for children. At present there are one-quarter to one-third million adults with insomnia every year. There are ten to twenty percent with severe depression, preventing

sleep. The adult patient rarely discusses insomnia with his doctor. The physician rarely asks about sleep habits or problems. (Latest information on insomnia from the West Vancouver Library, April 2003)

6. Pure water is necessary in order to remove toxins and create normal balance in the body. Water from the tap has to be purified by distillation because of the heavy metals and chemicals used in conventional filtration systems.

7. Fasting and detoxification of the many toxins in the body is essential in today's world. Fasting is done under careful supervision once or twice yearly, if necessary. Fasting institutions are listed for those interested.

8. Fresh air is important and to walk as often as possible in a park, where there are flowers and greenery, is beneficial for the lungs and circulation, as well as the heart.

9. Sunlight supports the planet and every living thing, including humans. It is necessary for growth, strong bones, and especially Vitamin D. Without Vitamin D, the body cannot supply adequate calcium. It is important not to tan in the heat of the day, but to be cautious and to sun in the early morning or late afternoon, and one-half hour at either time is sufficient to attain all the nutrients that the sun provides. The sun is not harmful, as Dr. Kime says in his book *Sunlight*. When one adequately supplies the body with good nutrition the skin is well protected, even without sunscreen.

10. To love oneself is to take care of the gift of life that has been bestowed to us. "Love is the striving for the

union of human souls … is the highest and only law of human life; and in the depth of his soul every human being – as we most clearly see in children – feels and knows this, he knows this until he is entangled by false teachings of the world." (Leo Tolstoy, *The Kingdom of God is Within You*, Farrar, Straus and Cudshy, 1961, p.10) When the human body is operating at its best, and every organ is functioning to its fullest capacity, an experience of true love of self and others, as well as the world, is felt every day. This love is manifested in living life to the fullest in one's creative productivity and service towards others and the community. To experience this emotion where peace abounds is the result of adhering to the simple laws of Nature, or God, and discontinuing the old life.

HEALTH AS A GIFT, VIRTUE, AND SCIENCE

Disease is a crisis, which means it is an effort on the part of the body to eliminate stored toxins. Disease is nature's way of curing. Pain is a friend, and messages the body gives through symptoms are to alert the individual that something needs to be changed. To suppress the symptoms pushes the problem further into the system, and the harmful chemicals in the form of drugs do not teach the patient how to remove the cause of disease.

In caring for the patient, a health care professional can solve the serious illnesses, as well as acute problems, by providing the conditions for health and eliminating harmful influences. This teaches the patient to be responsible for the gift of life by taking care of health. All pathological conditions and diseases, and tendencies to diseases, are the result of the transgression of the laws of human life.

The True Health Care System understands and promotes the basic cause of disease and teaches prevention. Health will be the outcome for all ages. Hospitals will become True Health Care Centers where fasting, detoxification, juice cleanses for those who cannot fast, and optimum dietary plans will be taught. Doctors will be teachers. Pharmaceuticals will be abolished and used only in cases of absolute emergency, i.e., accidents and unfortunate traumas. Pharmacies will be replaced with education centers based on nutritional needs of the human body. Dentists and doctors will be necessary for accidental-type work only. Insurance companies would be available for accidental-type of work also. Health education will be available at all community centers, as well as at schools and universities.

Libraries will have an adequate supply of books relating to the True Health Care System. Books, pamphlets, tapes, videos, and DVDs will be available for research and information by experts in the field of the Caring System. Medical colleges will be taught by health care professionals. As medical institutions begin to teach the facts about nutrition and the basic physiological and psychological needs of the body, fewer doctors, nurses, druggists, morticians, and staff working in pathology will be required. Teachers and educators, with qualified degrees in their field, will be in demand.

To solve the severe health care crisis means to let go of the past techniques of curing, and to teach the new method of caring for the sick. Sickness never comes without a cause, but it is always the consequence of violation to natural human laws. This system of health education promotes purification, vivification, and rejuvenation of the whole body. This is the science of caring for the patient. Hippocrates' saying, "Do no harm, and do not interfere with the doctor within," will be lived.

It is of grave concern that disease is costing nations around the world billions of dollars yearly, yet people are suffering, diseased, and dying prematurely. Children are dying of aids and cancer. What care is offered for a better life for anyone? Thomas Jefferson said, "If the people are given light they will find their own way." Individuals are prevented from receiving illumination as the health care system fails to educate and teach the basic principles of living in accordance with the natural laws that apply to human physiology. This is health in a nutshell. It is uncomplicated, and it is based on the physiological requirements of the human organism.

"The ways or processes by which the sick recover, when they do recover, no matter what the name given to the disease, or what the treatment employed, are strictly biological processes and are not susceptible of imitation or duplication by the practitioners of any school or so called healing. The forces and processes of the living organism alone restore health and these processes and operations are always in obedience to the same general principles of life; the power and the process by which the organism is developed and maintained are the same by which wounds are healed and health restored in disease." (Shelton, *Getting Well*, p. 7) In other words, healing is accomplished by the lawful and orderly operations of the same forces and processes that brought the organism into existence.

Dr. Ralph Cinque, who operates a fasting clinic in Texas, says this about the role one plays of being a patient:

"We surrender our dignity as rational beings when we place our health in the hand of physicians. We shackle ourselves, like peasants to a feudal lord, when we undergo a series of treatments. No intelligent self-respecting man or woman will feel comfortable as a participant in this degrading ritual. Assuming the role of 'patient' is unwholesome ... it entails admission of ignorance, ineptitude, and dependence. It evinces lack of self-knowledge ... a modern form of slavery." ("Human Dignity," *Health Science*, Nov. 1986)

Dr. Robert Mendelsohn, M.D., an established doctor who practiced in Illinois for many years and wrote several books on this subject says this of orthodox medicine: "I do not believe in Modern Medicine. I am a medical heretic. My aim is to persuade you to become a heretic too … I believe that despite all the super technology and elite bedside manner that's supposed to make you feel about as well cared for as an astronaut on the way to the moon, the greatest danger to your health is the doctor who practices Modern Medicine. I believe that Modern Medicine's treatments for disease are seldom effective, and that they're often more dangerous than the diseases they are designed to treat. I believe that more than ninety percent of Modern Medicine could disappear from the face of the earth – doctors, hospitals, dugs and equipment – and the effect on our health would be immediate and beneficial." Robert S. Mendelsohn, M.D., *Confessions of a Medical Heretic*, Contemporary Books, Chicago, Illinois, 1979, p. x)

STATISTICS

From the World Health Organization, Geneva, Switzerland, 2002, these are the following deaths:

Respiratory 3,560
Chronic Obstructive Pulmonary disease 2,672
Digestive diseases 1,987
Suicide 1,594
Cardiovascular disease 16,585
Ischaemic heart disease 7,181
Communicable disease 18,374
Malignant neoplasm 7,115
Cerebrovascular disease 5,454
Infectious and parasitic disease 10,937
Aids 2,866

In 2001

Aids 88,429
Aids, Africa alone 12,513

High child and very high adult 54,947
Nutritional deficiencies 32,988
Alzheimer – dementias 12,437
Suicide 48,802

500,000 have died from unsafe injection practices in a medical setting

The new Health Care System will reduce the risks of so many deaths and promote a healthy life. Dr. Hal Gunn reports 18,000 new cancer cases in British Columbia, Canada, alone. Colorectal cancer is the second leading cause of cancer-related deaths in North America. There are 500,000 to one million cases in America of reflex sympathetic dystrophy, a neurological condition, where the muscles and bones are eaten away and the patient loses mobility in six weeks; as the disease enters the spine the patient becomes an invalid. (Dr. Hal Gunn's Lecture, April 2003)

A woman in Vancouver, B.C., Canada, cashed in $7,000 of her savings to give toward the medical care without success. She now asks for help so she can attend a Chicago Clinic that asks for $35,000 to save her from becoming an invalid. (*Vancouver Sun* newspaper, May 12, 2003)

The statistics give us another clue as to the need for prevention and a new Health Care System, whereby patients and health seekers are taught that health care is self-care, and the power of healing is found within. The suppression of disease and symptoms may give temporary relief but has not taught the patient how to remove the cause of the disease and to restore health. Germs, viruses, diseases, and degeneration require a certain environment in which to grow, and they thrive in un-eliminated excrement that only fasting can rectify.

People are poisoned from retained waste created because of the violation of the natural laws.

Dr. Galor Matt, in his new book, *When the Body Says No*, says, "Emotional competence is necessary for good health ... how we live our lives in the fullest sense physically and emotionally, has an effect on our health." (*Vancouver Sun*, May 13, 2003, p. 12) Dr. Matt has noticed that cancer, chronic fatigue, colitis, Crohn's disease, and multiple sclerosis are diseases that manifest themselves in people who cannot say no, and cannot express anger. He also says these people need to learn self-acceptance and assertiveness in their personal and emotional copying style. A health support program will teach emotional poise as a prerequisite to optimum health.

Recently a young woman, twenty-one years of age, was committed to the local hospital for what she described as a mild case of colitis, which had troubled her for four months. After being at the hospital for two months and given great quantities of medication, including prednisone, she came home after much pleading with the medical establishment, with a serious case of colitis, as well as a severe case of depression. She tried to improve her nutritional habits and discontinue the medication with her doctor's help, who did not like the idea, but the withdrawal symptoms and the depression were too much with which to cope. The fear and anxiety prevented her from healing, and her doctor advised her that the best he could do for her was to remove her colon and then all bleeding would cease. She resorted to this and came home with a bag attached to her side, and although she had not stopped bleeding she now had another problem. She found it too difficult to cope with this tragedy, and jumped off a local bridge to end her misery.

As one can see from the above statistics, suicide is prevalent all over the world. The complications from drugs are physically, mentally and emotionally challenging. Although fasting has helped many colitis patients, they must be supervised carefully by an experienced professional.

The removal of organs and the suppression of symptoms does

not create health. There is no drug that can cure disease because it does not remove the cause of it. To ignore cause and effect portrays a lack of insight into the needs of the patient. Dr. Tilden, in his book on children, says, "A cold is elimination of toxin. To stop the symptoms means to stop elimination, which means to force the organism to retain the toxins and gradually grow a larger toleration, until life is overwhelmed by a so-called acute disease, or a chronic organic disease, which may end in the destruction of some important organ, or life itself." (Dr John Tilden, M.D., *Children, Their Health and Happiness*, 1960, p. 9)

Dr. Tilden used no medicine but practiced his theory of clearing the body of toxic poison and then allowing nature to make the cure, teaching his patients how to live so as not to create a toxic condition and to retain a healthy body freed of disease. To his patients he was "friend and mentor."

Education is the key to caring for the patient. No longer will the doctor have to treat disease but will teach the patient how to prevent it, and fasting will be the prescription, not medication. In order for a doctor to help the patient, the basic physiological and psychological needs of the human organism for life and health are required to be taught. Teachers at all schools will teach physiology as part of the health and science subjects so students will learn at a young age how to care for the body.

"The people need to learn that the natural condition of human beings is one of health and that every instance of sickness and suffering, unless caused by accident, is caused by some wrongdoing, either on the part of the sufferer or others." (Harriet N. Austin, M.D., reprinted in *Health Science*, 1985, p. 22|

The health care facilitator, doctor, nurse, or educator will teach each individual to be responsible for his or her health. Sickness never comes without a cause but is the consequence of violation of nature's laws, which regulate the human constitution. For instance, nature indicates the night for sleep, yet stimulants and food are taken instead.

The new Health Care System will provide opportunities for individuals to form chapters all over the world so that education and learning will be available for everyone.

The mission of the new Health Care System is to promote, educate, and inspire true health, which will benefit every person and the environment. This integrated education system will create health care professionals, counselors, and instructors who CARE.

The Eagle

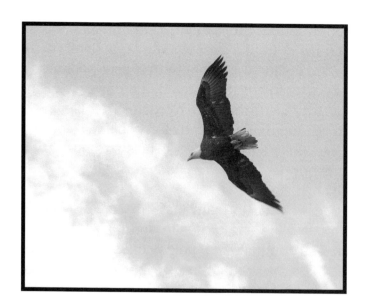

Strength - Power - Courage

CHAPTER VI

CONCLUSION

Shamrock/Four-leaf Clover

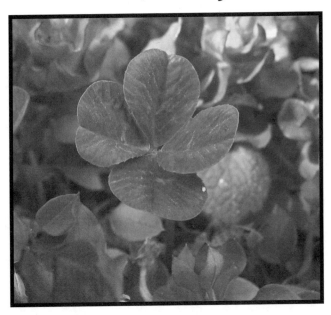

Good Fortune – Health – Achievement

"We have nothing to fear from knowledge, but from
ignorance everything"
– Dr. Joel Shew, M.D.

"Know thyself" is a saying that has been reiterated by the Greek Philosophers and sages throughout history to the present time. The human being is innately endowed with instinct, and primal humans relied upon supplying the basic needs of existence as the requisite to continued life. These needs are the same in health and disease. Healing is a biological process and its success depends upon simple, normal things of existence and not upon harmful substances. The individual who violates the laws of life cannot escape the consequences of such violation by taking a pill.

The human body is designed to live in good health for a lifetime, without pain, suffering, and premature death. The universal and immutable laws of self-preservation are based upon physiology and science. The successful power of self-healing that is intrinsic and possessed by every human being does not depend upon a new cure, but upon a vital power that has been with each human being from the beginning of existence.

In 2002 the Canadian Federal Government spent $3 billion on health care. Yet, prevention and care of the patient was not taught. In 2002, $1 billion was spent in Canada on health care. (Canadian Institution for Health Information, *Health Care Annual Report*, 2002)

In the year 2000, $1.3 trillion was spent in the United States on health care. (*New York Times*, Nov. 11, 2001, "Health Care May Reign Near Term," Kaiser family founder, www.org.) Statistics Canada, 2001 Annual Report: $2.5 billion was spent on mass media ads for drugs and $132 billion on drugs. The new cures, drugs, and remedies provided by new research and technology have not solved the serious health care problem, nor have they provided knowledge, education, and comfort or care for the sick. The *New York Times* reported recently that nearly 2.5 million unnecessary operations are performed in the United States each year, at a cost of $8 billion and result in over 12,000 needless deaths.

The fear of mad cow disease, SARS virus, and West Nile virus is being felt around the world today. Media reports suggest that "the public health system was too fragile and balkanized to effectively respond to the SARS crisis in Toronto" (*Vancouver Sun*, May 23, 2003, p. A19), and that SARS "perhaps was transported through extra-terrestrial microbes, missed through the atmosphere." (The Medical Journal, The "Lancet," *Vancouver Sun*, May 23, 2003). One can anticipate no hope for future epidemics. As the health care system continues to look to extrinsic factors as the cause of disease, a valid plan of care for the well and the sick is urgently needed.

A concerned senior research scientist for a large pharmaceutical company and author states his concern: "I, and others, suggested that the province's medical school include a course in iatrogenic medicine, something other countries had already done. Iatrogenic medicine is the study of harm done by treatment. Advocates of this proposal are still waiting. In the meantime, preventable errors are happening, and, as a result, patients are made ill, or die." (*North Shore News*, May 25, 2003, p. 8)

The human symptoms of sickness are nature's warning signal that action, not suppression, must be taken. Health care systems, schools of medicine, nursing schools, doctors, and old-age facilities treat the symptoms of disease with pharmaceuticals, which create side effects, harmful and dangerous to the patient. To remove the cause of disease and supply all of the conditions of health, as well as eliminate all harmful influences, is to be the basic teaching to replace the old mode of curing. This integral and valid plan of care, instead of cure, both of the well and of the sick, must be normal to life and have its roots in life itself.

Fasting demystifies the cause of illness by eliminating stored excrement, which is the primary cause of disease. The new Health Care system will educate rather than medicate. Fasting is the only remedial practice that conquers disease and helps the body restore and maintain optimum health. Fasting is Nature's remedy, as it rejuvenates, body, mind, and spirit and transforms life.

The physician with his knife, who believes that disease can be cured and remedied without removing the cause, has not understood cause and effect and portrays a lack of insight and care for the patient's true needs.

The new Health Care system goes back to the first physician, Hippocrates, 400 BC, whose oath was "Do no harm" and "The true physician is within," and will provide worldwide scientific health education. This new valid plan of care will solve the severe health care crisis and save billions of dollars for the world. It will teach that illness never comes without a cause but as a result of violating the laws of nature. With the power of knowledge and education, health will be restored, as well as the quality of life, and it will be possible to live so as to eliminate disease and suffering.

The human body is governed by natural law – God's Law – just as the moon, earth, sun, and stars. There is order in the universe and in the human organism, as the basic needs provide for a way of life. The basis of health is a natural condition, but the basis of disease is impaired function, yet both require the same basic needs. Symptoms are vital action as the body tries to return to homeostasis.

Health is a gift and virtue that requires diligence and perseverance. The advantage and value of the human body operating to its full capacity, and every cell, tissue and organ functioning normally, are powerful, constructive and creative, not only for self, but for the environment, the world, and everyone that we influence.

This body, the temple of love, is to be kept pure and holy, even though one day it may desert you, yet will leave an indelible magnetism resonating the True Health Care, which reflects that the human organism is a masterpiece of design capable of miracles.

Fasting creates the only valid means of restoring and maintaining optimum health. Fasting transforms the physical, mental, emotional, and spiritual human being. Fasting is an experience in self-awareness and elevates the human being to revere the sacredness of self and life and to create wholeness and fulfillment.

Illness comes as a teacher and messenger that one must address.

As I was praying for the healing of my baby I was directed to seek and find answers for myself. It was with an open mind and heart that I located Dr. Shelton's book, "*The Hygienic Care of Children*", shortly after—a Godsend. Learning that a change of lifestyle was necessary before the child could be well was something that did not come to mind, nor recommended by doctors.

The child's symptoms and physical condition were blessings and now we could take responsibility for his health and listen to his body.

Fasting on water only helps to promote transformation. Each individual must ask: What do I need to learn from this illness? It is a tool for change and it is a good thing. Consider, comprehend, and co-operate with the human body and do not interfere with healing.

It takes courage and strength to know oneself and to listen to the body.

Have patience, trust and faith in the powerful innate healing wisdom of the body.

Be transformed to wholeness by the renewal of your life.

Let us create health and let it begin with me.

When you stop eating, you become strong.

Fasting is healing.

And you will be like a flowered garden like a flowing spring whose waters never run dry.
— Isaiah 58:12

Chrysanthemum

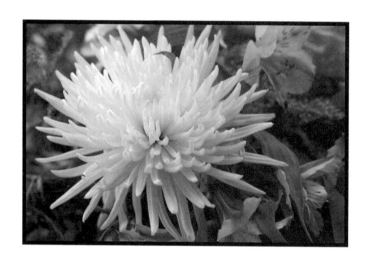

Truth – Hope – Longevity

"Beauty and Vitality are gifts from Nature
for those who live by her laws."
— Leonardo da Vince

SUMMARY

The Dove

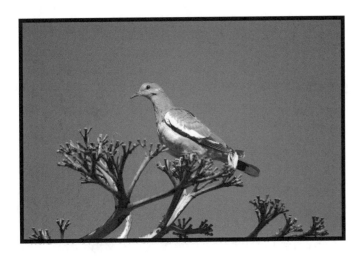

Peace - Forgiveness - Reassurance

The path to wholeness

Health is a state of soundness and integrity of organism, vigor efficiency of function, and excellence of mental functions.

The lifestyle suggested in this book as the most optimum is in coherence with Nature's laws. It is complete, total, and an all-encompassing way of living. It takes into consideration the mind, the body, and the spirit, both in health and disease. It requires individual responsibility and sensitive awareness of each area of life. There is no aspect of living from which it is excluded. It is the grand total of all life's expressions, here, now and beyond the mind. It is not only food and the physical; it is much more.

To be healthy is one of the most important gifts one can give to oneself, our children, our family and the world. It is also a way of expressing gratitude for life itself. A healthy body manifests itself in a healthy mind, emotional health, and a spiritual life. A healthy individual can go into the world and be a channel of grace in many areas of life and work. In helping others use the gifts and talents inherent within, we will empower our lives and others with the greatest achievement: to reach fulfillment and conquer the fear of pain and suffering.

Healing transcends everything that may be disrupting the body, mind, or Spirit. Each one can now become who they were meant to be.

I wrote this book so you could find a simple solution to attain perfect health for the rest of your life. First and foremost: What does your body NEED to be healthy is what you may ask? Do you need a drug? No, it is not the lack of a drug that has made you ill. Or, why am I sick? You need to know the physical, mental, emotional and spiritual needs of your body. You need to nurture your body with fresh air, clean water, whole, live, plant-based quality foods, emotional poise, sunlight, rest, sleep, relaxation; to fast and cleanse your body, mind and spirit, to be productive and to love and take care of this gift of life, as well as to have loving relationships.

As I searched and prayed for healing of my son's health problems, I found a sympathetic doctor, as was the first physician, Hippocrates, who taught, informed and inspired me with the basic truths of health. I have documented all these truths in this book; and you need to make note of every page in this book and make it your blueprint for feeling good, looking great with vibrant energy, for the rest of your life.

To live passionately and purposefully you need to be healthy. This simple approach to perfect health will give you peace, joy and freedom. It is time to go back to ancient times to celebrate good health by removing the cause of illness, supplying the conditions for health and experience the healing power of Nature inherent within. Listen, be still and nurture the physical mental emotional, intellectual, and spiritual being so "fearfully and wonderfully" made, to last a lifetime!

"Two roads diverged in a wood and I -
I took the one less traveled by.
And that has made all the difference"
– Robert Frost

Health and strength are better than any gold.

BIBLIOGRAPHY

Barnard, Neal, M.D. "Good Medicine." From CFRM, Vol. XII. (2003).

Bragg, Paul C. "Build Powerful Nerve Force." *Health Science*. Santa Barbara, CA.

Buchinger, Otto H.F., M.D. *About Fasting, A Royal Road To Healing*. Thorsons Publisher Ltd., England. (1961).

Cott, Allan, M.D. *Fasting: The Unlimited Diet*. Bantum Books. (August 1979).

_____. *Fasting As a Way of Life*. Bantum Books. (May 1977).

Fuhrman, Joel, M.D. *Fasting and Eating for Health*. First St. Martin's Griffin Edition. (May 1998)

Gian-Cursio, Christopher. *Eternal Health Truths of a Century Ago*. Hygean Press, Woodside, NY. (1960).

Graham, Sylvester, M.D. *Lectures On The Science of Human Life*. Fowler & Wells, Publishers, NY. (1980).

Mendelsohn, Robert S., M.D. *Confessions of A Medical Heretic*. Contemporary Books Inc., Chicago, IL. (1979).

Rasmus, Alsaker, M.D. "The Cause and Cure of all Disease." Reprinted from *Health Culture*.

Ryan, Thomas. *Fasting Rediscovered*. Paulist Press, NY. (1981).

Shelton, H.M. *Superior Nutrition*. Dr. Shelton's Health School, Publisher. (1951-2003).

_____. *The Original Natural Hygiene Weight Loss Diet Book*. Keats Publishing, Inc. (1986).

_____. *The Science and Fine Art of Fasting*. Chicago Natural Hygiene Press. (1978).

_____. *Health for the Millions*.

_____. *The Hygiene System, Vol. I, Orthobionomics*.

_____. *Man's Pristine Way of Life*. Dr. Shelton's Health School. San Antonio, TX. (1968).

_____. *Getting Well*. Health Research, CA.

_____. *Health for All*. Health Research, Mokelumne Hill, CA.

_____. *The Hygienic System, Vol. III, Orthotrophy*. Dr. Shelton's Health School, Publisher, San Antonio, TX. (1934).

_____. *Rubies In The Sand*. (1961).

Dr. Shelton's Hygienic Reviews and Educators. (1979-80).

Sinclair, Upton. *The Fasting Cure*. Los Angeles, CA. (1923).

Shew, Joel, M.D. *Children in Health and Disease*. Fowlers and Wells Publishers, NY. (1852).

Thayer, Gilbert. *Health for One Hundred Years*. The National Health Bureau, LaFayette, IN.

Tilden, John H., M.D. *Toxemia Explained, The Basic Cause of all Disease*. Denver, CO. (1926).

Trall, Russell T. *The True Healing Art*. Fowler & Wells, NY. (February 12, 1862).

Willard, Jo. *The Journals of Natural Hygiene*. Huntington, CT. (1988-98).

Grapes

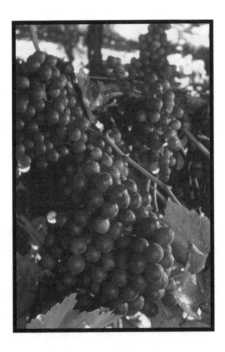

Revitalization – Sustenance – Youthfulness

About the Author

Halanna Matthew, is a Doctor of Health Science, who specializes in prevention, nutrition and restoring health. Born in Manitoba, Canada, now works in Vancouver, BC Canada, graduated from several universities, has studied the Alexander Technique, and has developed courses on Effective Weight Loss, Childrens' Health, Cancer, Heart Disease, etc. Has researched all diseases and presently works at universities, schools, and with individuals teaching optimum health.

Dr. Matthew is author of "Physical Mental and Spiritual Health, and is completing a manuscript, *"Perfect Palette"*.

Dr. Matthew hosted a radio program, "Dynamic Health" and has created programs for universities, schools and institutions on Effective Weight Loss, The Best Nutrition, How to Age Gracefully and many other subjects. Future radio programs and tv education programs will be available.

With over 25 years experience, educating people Dr. Matthew continues effective counselling and education based on tried and true methods acquired from years of knowledge and experience.